Health Care Administration:

A Selected Bibliography

Health Care Administration:

A Selected Bibliography

SAMUEL LEVEY, *Ph.D.*

Professor and Director, Graduate Program in Health Care Administration, Baruch College—Mount Sinai School of Medicine, City University of New York

N. PAUL LOOMBA, *Ph.D.*

Professor and Chairman, Department of Management, Baruch College, City University of New York

J. B. Lippincott Company
Philadelphia · Toronto

ISBN-0-397-52060-3

Library of Congress Catalog Card Number 72—11486

Printed in the United States of America

3   2   1

Library of Congress Cataloging in Publication Data

Levey, Samuel.
    Health care administration: a selected bibliography.

    Companion vol. to Health care administration: a managerial
perspective.
    1. Public health administration—Bibliography.
I. Loomba, Narendra Paul, 1927-   joint author.
II. Title.
Z6673.L47   016.658'91'3621   72-11486
ISBN-0-397-52060-3

DEDICATED TO

The Managers of Health Care Systems

Exhibit A.   Organization of the Book

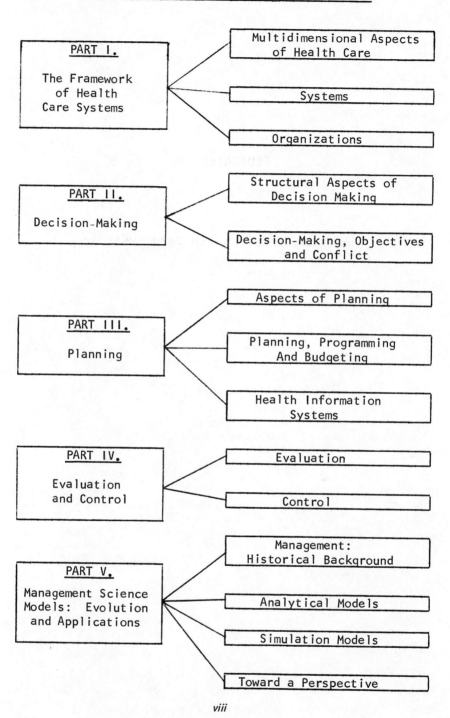

PREFACE

This bibliography is a companion volume to our
main book entitled: <u>Health Care Administration: A</u>
<u>Managerial Perspective</u> (Philadelphia, Pa.: J. B. Lippincott
Company, 1973). A schematic presentation of the organization of the main book is shown in Exhibit A. The main book
is organized into fourteen chapters, which cover a very
broad spectrum of management concepts, methods, tools and
techniques. Its contents were selected and organized with
the overall objective of providing pragmatic approaches to
the resolution of managerial problems in health organizations. This bibliography represents an additional effort
for achieving the same overall objective.

We decided to publish the bibliography as a
separate volume primarily for two reasons. First, it was
impossible to compress into one volume all the available
and relevant material encompassed by the full scope of
various topics that we have included in the main book. Yet,
we felt strongly that once the reader has been exposed to
the nature, structure, properties, and application potential of various management topics, he ought also be provided
with access to additional sources related to theory as well
as practice. In order to achieve this purpose, we divided

the bibliography into fourteen parts--corresponding to the fourteen chapters of the main book. Each part of the bib-liography,therefore, is in support of the corresponding chapter in the main book, and contains reference materials for further study and research. The second reason for publishing the bibliography as a separate volume stems from the fact that the rate of publication in the fields of management and health administration is increasing very rapidly. If the managers of health institutions are to be kept aware of the most useful, relevant, and meaningful new publications, a mechanism which can update the "state of the art" with an optimum frequency must be found. A selected bibliography which can be kept current provides such a mechanism. The bibliography, as a separate volume, is tied to the main book conceptually and contentwise—yet its revision can be effected independently.

Any classification attempt must strike a com-promise between the dangers of drawing arbitrary boundary lines on the one hand and suffering from redundancy on the other (in the sense of the same elements being found in different classifications). Whenever such a dilemma was faced by us, we chose redundancy for the sake of economy of time. In the interest of convenience for the user, some entries appearing in the main book were also included in this volume.

We plan to update the bibliography every two years, and will expand its scope as we gain more experience. To this purpose, we encourage our readers to write to us directly, and we will utilize their suggestions in the next revision.

We would like to thank our graduate students for their help and assistance in completing the bibliography project. We are especially indebted to Mr. Harjinder Singh of Computer Design Corporation who coordinated the entire project and worked very diligently for long hours. Mrs. Lynette Robinson typed the manuscript, gathered important items of information to complete several entries, and served as a valuable research associate. We also appreciate the support and encouragement of Linda Levey and Mary Loomba. The idea of publishing the bibliography as a separate volume originated from Mary Loomba, who is Head of the Division of Reader Services at the College of New Rochelle.

Samuel Levey
N. Paul Loomba

New York, N.Y.

C O N T E N T S

Part 1.

MULTIDIMENSIONAL ASPECTS OF HEALTH CARE

American Hospital Association, Classification of Health
   1968   Care Institutions: Chicago, Ill.

American Medical Association, Distribution of Physicians
   1971   in the United States, 1970, Center for Health
        Services Research and Development: Chicago,Ill.

Ammer, D.S., "Recognizing Economic Indicators," Hospital
   1969   Progress, vol. 50, October, pp. 25-29.

Anderson, J.M., "The HUB of Health Care," Hospital Progress,
   1967   October, pp. 100-104.

Anderson, O.W., The Uneasy Equilibrium, New Haven, Conn.:
   1968   College and University Press.

Anderson, O.W., "Universal and Compulsory Health Insurance:
   1970   The Last Alternative," Hospital Administration,
        vol. 15, no. 3, Summer, pp. 35-53.

Archives of Environmental Health, "Need to Improve Delivery
   1968   of Health Services," vol. 16, May, pp. 699.

Arnold, M.,et al., Administering Health Systems: Issues
   1971   and Perspectives, New York: Aldine Atherton.

Bakke, G.S., "Dimensions of the Health Care Crisis,"
   1970   Hospital Progress, vol. 51, April, pp. 50-53.

Balknap, I. and J.G. Steinle, The Community and Its Hospi-
   1963   tals, Syracuse, N.Y.: Syracuse University Press.

Bamberger, L., "Opportunities for Official Health Agencies
   1966   in the Community Action Program," American
        Journal of Public Health, vol. 56, April, pp.
        596-602.

Bauer, R.A., The Study of Policy Formation, N.Y.: Free
   1968   Press.

Beloff, J.S. and E.R. Weinerman, "Yale Studies in Family
1967   Health Care: Planning and Pilot-testing of a
        New Program," <u>Journal of the American Medical
        Association</u>, vol. 199, February, pp. 383-389.

Bennett, I.L., "The Scientific and Educational Basis for
1970   Medical Care," Unpublished paper presented at
        New York Health Services Research and Policy
        Seminar, Dec. 1, p. 2.

Bennis, W.G., et al., <u>The Planning of Change</u>, New York:
1969   Holt, Rinehart and Winston, Inc.

Berke, M. and J.A. Hahn, "Health Care in the 1970's. What
1970   are the Issues?" <u>Hospitals</u>, vol. 44, January 1,
        pp. 46-51.

<u>Blue Cross and Blue Shield Fact Book</u>, Chicago, Ill.: Blue
1971   Cross Association, p. 4.

Blum, H.L. and G.M. Keranen, <u>Control of Chronic Diseases in
1966   Man</u>, New York: The American Public Health Assoc.

Boulding, K.E., "Ecology and Environment," <u>Trans-Action</u>,
1970   March, pp. 38-44.

Brenner, M.H. and E.R. Weinerman, "An Ambulatory Service
1969   Data System," <u>American Journal of Public Health</u>,
        vol. 59, July, pp. 1154-1168.

Brown, M., "An Economic Analysis of Hospital Operations,"
1970   <u>Hospital Administration</u>, vol. 15, Spring, pp.
        60-74.

Brown, R.E., "The Hospital: Proper Portal to All Health
1969   Care," <u>Hospital Physician</u>, May, vol. 5, pp.
        143, 146-147.

Brown, R.E., "Health Care Issues in the 1970's. Changing
1970   Management and Corporate Structure," <u>Hospitals</u>,
        vol. 44, January, pp. 77-83.

Business Week, "The $60-billion Crisis Over Medical Care,"
    1970   January 17, pp. 50-64.

Business Week, "What Controls Mean to Medical Care,"
    1972   January 1, pp. 38-39.

Chamberlain, J., et al., "The Population Served by the Out-
    1966   patient Department of a London Teaching Hospi-
            tal: A Study of Guys," Medical Care, vol. 4,
            April-June, pp. 81-88.

Cohen, W.J., "National Health Insurance--Problems and Pros-
    1970   pects," Michael M. Davis Lecture, Center for
            Health Administration Studies, University of
            Chicago.

Crosby, E.L., "Health Care Issues in the 1970's, Hospitals
    1970   as the Center of Health Care Universe,"Hospitals,
            vol. 44, January 1, pp. 52-56.

Curran, W.J., "Public Health and the Law," American Journal
    1969   of Public Health, vol. 59, May, pp. 854-855.

Davies, R.L., "Facilities and Equipment for Health Services,"
    1966   Milbank Memorial Fund Quarterly, vol. 49, Part
            2, July, pp. 266-268.

Deland, E.C. and B. Waxman, "Technological Opportunities
    1969   for the Delivery of Health Care," Proceedings
            of the Institute of Electrical and Electronics
            Engineers, IEEE, vol. 57, November, pp.
            1842-1845.

Densen, P., et al., "Primary Medical Care for an Urban
    1968   Population: A Survey of Present and Potential
            Utilization," Journal of Medical Education,
            vol. 43, December, pp. 1244-1249.

Derwinski, E.J., "We Need More Doctors," Congressional
    1969   Record, vol. 115, May 5, p. E3622.

Devey, G.B., "Toward Automated Health Services," <u>Proceed-</u>
   1969   <u>ings of the IEEE</u>, vol. 57, November, pp. 1828-
           1842.

<u>Dollars and Sense</u>, A Study Report for the W.K. Kellogg
   1971   Foundation, Battle Creek, Michigan, October.

Dressler, F.G.,Jr., <u>Patient Care Assessment in Extended</u>
   1971   <u>Health Care Facilities</u>, New Haven, Conn.:
           Connecticut Health Services Research Series.

Drucker, P.F., <u>The Age of Discontinuity: Guidelines to our</u>
   1968   <u>Changing Society</u>, New York: Harper & Row.

Dubos, R.J., <u>So Human An Animal</u>, New York: Scribner.
   1968

Dunlop, J.T., "Some Facets of the Economics of Health Care
   1970   Delivery," <u>Journal of Medical Education</u>, vol.
           45, March, pp. 133-138.

Durbin, R.L. and G. Antelman, "A Study of the Effects of
   1964   Selected Variables on Hospital Utilization,"
           <u>Hospital Management</u>, vol. 98, August, pp. 57-60.

<u>Earnings of Hospital Employees in New York State</u>, 1957-
   1969   1968, New York: State Department of Health,
           October.

Ehrenreich, B. and J. Ehrenreich, <u>The American Health</u>
   1970   <u>Empire</u>, N.Y.: Random House.

Eilers, R.D., "National Health Insurance: What Kind and
   1971   How Much," <u>The New England Journal of Medi-</u>
           <u>cine</u>, vol. 284, April 22, pp. 881-886.

Elling, R.H., <u>National Health Care</u>, New York: Aldine-
   1971   Atherton.

Engle, R.L.,Jr., "Medical Diagnosis: Present, Past,Future.
    1963   Philosophical Foundation and Historical Develop-
             ment of Our Concepts of Health, Disease, and
             Diagnosis," Archives of Internal Medicine, vol.
             112, October, pp. 520-529.

Fein, R., The Doctor Shortage, Washington, D.C.: The
    1967   Brookings Institute.

Feldstein, M.S., The Rising Cost of Hospital Care, Washing-
    1971   ton, D.C.: Information Resources Press.

Feldstein, P.J., "Research on Demand for Health Services,"
    1967   Milbank Memorial Fund's Health Services Research,
             edited by D. Mainland, N.Y.: The Fund, pp.
             128-165.

Feldstein, P.J., "Applying Economic Concepts to Hospital
    1968   Care," Hospital Administration, vol. 13,
             Winter, pp. 68-89.

Ferkiss, V.C., Technological Man, New York: Braziller.
    1969

Financial Requirements of Health Care Institutions and Ser-
    1969   vices, Statement of, Chicago, Ill.: American
             Hospital Association.

Flagle, C.D., "Viewpoints," Health Services Research, vol.
    1969   4, Spring, pp. 6-13.

Flagle, C.D., "Technological Development in the Health Ser-
    1969   vices," Proceedings of the IEEE, vol. 57, Nov-
             ember, pp. 1847-1852.

Forsyth, G. and R.F.L.Logan, The Demand for Medical Care,
    1960   published for the Nuffield Provincial Hospitals
             Trust, London: Oxford University Press.

Fortune Magazine, "Our Ailing Medical System," January, pp.
    1970   79-99.

Fortune Magazine, "It's Time to Operate," January.
    1970

Freidson, E., Professional Dominance: The Social Structure
1970   of Medical Care, N.Y.: Atherton Press, Inc.

Fuchs, V.R., "The Contribution of Health Services to the
1966   American Economy," Milbank Memorial Fund Quarterly, vol. 49, October, pp. 65-103.

Fuchs, V.R., "Basic Forces Influencing Cost of Medical Care,"
1967   in Report of the National Conference on Medical
Costs, National Conference on Medical Costs,
Washington, D.C., June 27, U.S. Dept. of HEW,
Government Printing Office.

Fuchs, V.R., "Medical Costs: Why They are What They are,"
1967   Modern Hospital, vol. 109, September, pp. 104-
114.

Fuchs, V.R., "The Growing Demand for Medical Care," The New
1968   England Journal of Medicine, July 25, vol. 279,
pp. 190-195.

Fuchs, V.R., "Improving the Delivery of Health Services,"
1969   The Journal of Bone and Joint Surgery, vol. 51-a,
March, pp. 407-412.

Galbraith, J.K., "Economics and the Quality of Life," En-
1965   counter, vol. 24, January, pp. 31-39.

Galbraith, J.K., The New Industrial State, Boston: Houghton
1967   Mifflin.

Gamm, S., Toward Collective Bargaining in Non-Profit Hospi-
1968   tals: Impact of New York Law, Bulletin 60,
Ithaca, N.Y.: New York State School of Industrial
and Labor Relations, Cornell University.

Gardner, J.W., "On the Individual and Society," Harvard
1969   Alumni Bulletin, May 19, pp. 31-34.

Gardner, J.W., "The 1970's, Time to Wake Up," presented at
1969   the National Press Club, Washington, D.C., December 9.

Geiger, H.J. and R.D. Cohen, "Trends in Health Care Delivery
1971   Systems," Inquiry, vol. 8, March, pp. 32-34.

Georgopoulos, B. and G. Wieland, Nationwide Study of Coordi-
1964   nation and Patient Care in Voluntary Hospitals,
        No. 2178, Ann Arbor, Michigan: Institute for
        Social Research.

Georgopoulos,B. and H.Aleksander, "The American General Hos-
1967   pital as a Complex Social System," Health Ser-
        vices Research, vol. 2, Spring, pp. 76-111.

Ginzberg, E., Urban Health Services, The Case of New York,
1971   N.Y.: Columbia University Press.

Goddard, J.L., "The Burden of Responsibility--The Govern-
1969   ment's Role," Archives of Environmental Health,
        vol. 18, February, pp. 249-253.

Greenwood, F. and C.R. Kendrick, "Computer Technology: A
1968   Challenge for Hospital Administrators," Hospital
        Administration, vol. 13, Summer, pp. 62-67.

Gue, R.L., "An Introduction to the Systems Approach in the
1969   Dietary Department," Hospitals, vol. 43, Septem-
        ber 1, pp. 100-101.

Guide Issue, Hospitals, Part Two, vol. 45, no. 15, August 1.
1971

Hagedorn, H. and J.J. Dunlop, "Health Care Delivery as a
1969   Social System: Inhibitions and Constraints on
        Change," Proceedings of the IEEE, vol. 57, Nov-
        ember, pp. 1894-1900.

Hagner, S.B., et al., "Patient Outcome in a Comprehensive
1968   Medical Clinic," Medical Care, vol. 6, March-
        April, pp. 144-156.

Hanft, R.S., "National Health Expenditures, 1950-1965,"
1967   Social Security Bulletin, vol. 3, Feb, pp. 3-13.

Hanlon, J.J., Principles of Public Health Administration,
1964   4th Edition, St. Louis: C.V.Mosby Co.

Health, Education and Welfare, Dept. of, <u>Health Manpower</u>
  1964   <u>Source Book</u>, Section 18, "Manpower in the 1960's"
          Public Health Service Pub. No. 263, Washington,
          D.C.: Government Printing Office.

Health, Education and Welfare, Dept. of; Public Health Ser-
  1965   vice, <u>Grants for Comprehensive Health Services</u>
          <u>for Children and Youth: Policies and Procedures</u>,
          Washington, D.C.: Government Printing Office.

Health, Education and Welfare, Dept. of; Public Health Ser-
  1965   vice, Social Security Administration, Div. of
          Research and Statistics, "National Ecpenditures
          for Health Care Purposes by Object of Expendi-
          tures and Source of Funds, 1960-1963," <u>Research</u>
          <u>and Statistics</u>, Note No. 10.

Health, Education and Welfare, Dept. of; Bureau of Health
  1967   Manpower, <u>Health Manpower Perspective</u>, PHS
          Publication No. 1667, Washington, D.C.: GPO.

Health, Education and Welfare, Dept. of; Public Health Ser-
  1969   vice, "The Nation's Health Care System," <u>Weekly</u>
          <u>Compilation of Presidential Documents</u>, vol. 5,
          July 14, 1969, pp. 963-969, (Washington, D.C.:
          Office of the Federal Registrar--National Arch-
          ives and Records Service.)

Health, Education and Welfare, Dept. of; Public Health Ser-
  1971   vice, <u>Health Resources Statistics, 1970</u>, Feb.

Health, Education and Welfare, Dept. of; Administration's
  1971   White Paper, <u>Towards A Comprehensive Health</u>
          <u>Policy for the 1970's</u>, May.

Health, Education and Welfare, Dept. of; <u>Medical Care Costs</u>
  1972   <u>and Prices: Background Book</u>, Social Security
          Administration.

Health Information Foundation, <u>An Inventory of Social and</u>
  1961   <u>Economic Research in Health</u>, 9th edition, 1960,
          10th edition, 1961, New York.

Health Insurance Data, Source Book, 1971-1972, New York:
1971   Health Insurance Institute.

Herman, M.W., "The Poor: The Medical Needs and the Health
1972   Services Available to Them," The Annals of the
American Academy of Political and Social Science,
vol. 399, January, pp. 12-21.

Higher Education and the Nation's Health, New York: Carnegie
1970   Commission on Higher Education.

Hill, L.A., "Financial Incentives: How Could They Reshape
1969   the Health Care System?" Hospitals, vol. 43,
June 16, pp. 58-62.

Hilleboe, H.E., "Public Health in the U.S. in the 1970's,"
1968   American Journal of Public Health, vol. 58,
September, pp. 1588-1610.

Hindle, A. and K. Alfred, "Computer Simulation--An Aid to
1969   Management and Planning," Hospital International,
vol. 3, June, pp. 21-23.

Historical Statistics of the United States, 1789-1945, U.S.
1949   Dept. of Commerce, Bureau of the Census, Washington, D.C.: Government Printing Office.

Horvath, W.J., "Need for Estimating the Influence of Tech-
1968   nological and Social Changes on Future Health
Facility Requirements," Health Services Research,
Spring, pp. 3-9.

Hospitals, "The Nation's Hospitals: A Statistical Profile,"
1971   Part 2, August.

Hospital Costs in New York State, Albany, New York: Hospi-
1969   tal Association of New York, August 1.

Howland, D., "The Development of a Methodology for the Eval-
1958   uation of Patient Care," Progress Reports, The
Engineering Experiment Station, Ohio State University, 1958, 1959, 1960.

Howland, D. and W.E. McDowell, "The Measurement of Patient
    1964   Care: A Conceptual Framework," Nursing Research,
            Winter, vol. 13, pp. 4-8.

Ingbar, M.L. and L.D. Taylor, Hospital Costs: A Case Study
    1967   of Massachusetts, Cambridge, Mass.: Harvard
            University Press.

James, G., "Fragmentation: Crucial Flow in the Health Care
    1964   Complex," Hospitals, vol. 38, November 1.

Jeffers, J.R., et al., "On the Demand Versus Need for Medi-
    1971   cal Services and the Concept of 'Shortage',"
            American Journal of Public Health, vol. 61, Jan.
            pp. 46-63.

Johns, R.J., "What is Blunting the Impact of Engineering on
    1969   Hospitals?" Proceedings of the IEEE, vol. 57,
            November, pp. 1823-1827.

Kahn, H. and A.J. Wiener, The Year 2000, New York: The
    1967   Macmillan Co.

Katz, A.H. and J.S. Felton, Health and the Community, N.Y.:
    1965   The Free Press.

Kaufman, H., "The Political Ingredients of Public Health
    1966   Services: A Neglected Area of Research," Mil-
            bank Memorial Fund Quarterly, vol. XLIV, October,
            pp. 13-34.

Kissick, W.L., "Forecasting Health Manpower Needs," Hospi-
    1967   tals, vol. 41, September 16, pp. 47-51.

Klarman, H.E., The Economics of Health, N.Y.: Columbia
    1965   University Press.

Knowles, J.H., "The Quantity and Quality of Medical Man-
    1969   power: A Review of Medicines' Current Efforts,"
            Journal of Medical Education, vol. 44, February,
            pp. 81-118.

Landgraf, W.E., "Needed: New Perspectives on Health Ser-
    1967   vices," Harvard Business Review, vol. 45, Sept.-
            Oct., pp. 75-83.

Leavell, H.R. and E.G. Clark, Preventive Medicine, N.Y.:
1958   McGraw-Hill Book Company.

Lee, P., "Health and Well Being, Some Dangers in Valid
1967   Social Measurement," Annals of the American
         Academy of Political and Social Sciences, vol.
         373, September, pp. 193-207.

Lentz, E., "Hospital Administration--One of a Species,"
1957   Administrative Science Quarterly, vol. 1, March,
         pp. 444-463.

Levey, S. and S.M. Lubow, "Survey of Long-term and Extended
1968   Care Facilities," Nursing Homes, vol. 17, May,
         pp. 27-30.

Lewis, I.J., "Government Investment in Health Care,"
1971   Scientific American, April, vol. 224, pp. 17-25.

Lindblom, C.E., The Policy Making Process, Englewood Cliffs,
1968   N.J.: Prentice-Hall.

Marston, R.Q., "To Meet the Nation's Health Needs," The
1968   New England Journal of Medicine, vol. 279,
         September 5, pp. 520-524.

Mattson, H.W., "Future Hospitals," International Science
1966   and Technology, no. 56, August, pp. 30-37.

Mauksch, H.O., "It Defies All Logic...But a Hospital Does
1960   Function," Modern Hospital, vol. 95, October,
         pp. 67-70.

McLachlan, G., Problems and Progress in Medical Care:
1964   Essays on Current Research, Nuffield Provincial
         Hospitals Trusts, London: Oxford University
         Press.

McMahon, B., et al., Epidemiologic Methods, Boston: Little,
1960   Brown & Co.

McNerney, W.J., "Comprehensive Personal Health Care Services:
1967   A Management Challenge to the Health Professions,"
         American Journal of Public Health, vol. 57,
         October, pp. 1717-1727.

McNerney, W.J., "The Health Administration Establishment:
    1969   Underachiever," American Journal of Public
            Health, vol. 59, October, pp. 1799-1808.

Mechanic, D., "Symposium: Trends in the Delivery of Health
    1971   Services," Inquiry, vol. 8, March, pp. 3-8.

Mechanic, D., "Human Problems and the Organization of Health
    1972   Care," The Annals of the American Academy of
            Political and Social Sciences, vol. 399, January,
            pp. 1-11.

Merriam, I.C., "Social Welfare Expenditures, 1964-1966,"
    1965   Social Security Bulletin, vol. 1, October, pp.
            3-16.

Mesthene, E.G., Technological Change, Cambridge, Mass.:
    1970   Harvard University Press.

Millis, J.S., A Rational Public Policy for Medical Education
    1971   and Its Financing, N.Y.: The National Fund for
            Medical Education.

Muller, H.J., The Children of Frankenstein, A Primer on
    1970   Modern Technology and Human Values, Bloomington,
            Indiana: Indiana University Press.

Mushkin, S.J., "Health as an Investment," Journal of Poli-
    1962   tical Economy, Supplement, vol. 70, October,
            pp. 129-157.

National Advisory Commission on Health Manpower, Report of;
    1967   Vol. 1 and 2, Washington, D.C.: U.S. Govern-
            ment Printing Office.

National Center for Health Statistics, Health Manpower and
    1968   Health Facilities, 1968, Public Health Service
            Publication No. 1509, Washington, D.C.: Govern-
            ment Printing Office.

National Commission on Community Health Services, Health is
    1966   a Community Affair, Cambridge, Mass: Harvard
            University Press.

"The Nation's Health Care System," Presidential Documents,
1969   vol. 5, July 14, pp. 963-969, Washington, D.C.:
         Office of the Federal Register-National Archives
         and Records Service.

Navarro, V., "Planning Personal Health Services: A Marko-
1969   vian Model," Medical Care, vol. 7, May-June,
         pp. 242-249.

Newhouse, J.P. and V. Taylor, "How Shall we Pay for Hospital
1971   Care?" The Public Interest, vol. 23, Spring,
         pp. 78-92.

New York Times, "U.S. Health Crisis Called Severe for Minor-
1971   ities," June 13.

New York Times, "Health Department to Monitor Cost Rise for
1971   Hospital Services," October 3, p. 79.

New York Times, "Computer is Used to Monitor Health of 150
1971   Teamsters," October 3, p. 71.

Nixon, President Richard M., State of the Union Address,
1972   January.

Odegaard, C.E., "Crises in American Health Care," Hospital
1969   Administration, vol. 14, Summer, pp. 67-80.

"The Plight of the U.S. Patient," Time, February 21, pp.
1969   53-58.

Pomrinse, S.D., "The Economics of Excellence in Medical Care,"
1971   Journal of the Association of Hospital Personnel
         Administrators, vol. 10, May, p. 5-9.

Rabin, D.L. and J.E.C. Walker, "Initial Patient Care Under
1967   Contrasting Clinic System (Abstract)," Clinical
         Research, vol. 15, April, p. 343.

Reder, M., "Some Problems in the Economics of Hospitals,"
1965   The American Economic Review, vol. 55, May, pp.
         472-492.

Reed, L.S. and M. Dwyer, <u>Health Insurance Plans, Other Than</u>
  1971   <u>Blue Shield or Blue Cross Plans or Insurance Com-</u>
       <u>panies, 1970 Survey</u>, Social Security Administra-
       tion, Research Report No. 35, Washington, D.C.:
       Government Printing Office.

Rein, M., <u>Social Policy: Issues of Choice and Change</u>, N.Y.:
  1970   Random House.

Revans, R.W., <u>Standards for Morale: Cause and Effect in</u>
  1964   <u>Hospitals</u>, Nuffield Provincial Hospitals Trust,
       London: Oxford University Press.

Ribicoff, Senator A., "The Healthiest Nation Myth," <u>Satur-</u>
  1970   <u>day Review</u>, August 22, pp. 18-20.

Rice, D.P., "Economic Value of Human Life," <u>American Journal</u>
  1967   <u>of Public Health</u>, vol. 57, November, pg. 1954.

Rice, D.P., "Estimating the Cost of Illness," <u>American</u>
  1967   <u>Journal of Public Health</u>, vol. 57, March, pp.
       424-439.

Rice, R., "An Analysis of the Hospital as an Economic Organ-
  1966   ism," <u>Modern Hospital</u>, vol. 106, April, pp.
       87-91.

Richart, R.H., et al., "Administrative Research and Develop-
  1964   ment," <u>Hospital Progress</u>, January, pp. 69-77.

Robertson, A., "Health Services and Education for the Health
  1967   Professions," <u>Medical Care</u>, vol. 5, March-April,
       pp. 75-77.

Robinson, G.H., et al., "Prediction of Hospital Length of
  1966   Stay," <u>Health Services Research</u>, vol. 1, Winter,
       pp. 287-300.

Roemer, M.I., "Teaching of Medical Care Administration:
  1966   Emerging Issues," <u>Medical Care</u>, vol. 4, January,
       pp. 60-62.

Roemer, M.I., A National Health System: Analysis and Pro-
  1969   jections," <u>Hospital Progress</u>, vol. 50, Septem-
       ber, pp. 71-75ff.

Rogatz, P., "Health Services in a Democracy," Bulletin of
1969   the Academy of Medicine, vol. 45, May, pp. 421-436.

Rogatz, P., "The Health Care System," Hospitals, vol. 44,
1970   April 16, pp. 47-50.

Rogers, E.S., Human Ecology and Health, N.Y.:   The Macmillan
1960   Company.

Roney, J.G., Jr., "A Case Study of Administrative Structure
1965   in a Health Department," Human Organization,
         vol. 24, Winter, pp. 346-352.

Rosner, M.W., "Economic Determinants of Organizational Inno-
1968   vation," Administrative Science Quarterly, vol.
         12, March, pp. 614-625.

Roy, Honorable W. R., speech of; in the House of Represen-
1971   tatives, November 11, Congressional Record.

Sade, R.M., "Medical Care as a Right: A Refutation," New
1971   England Journal of Medicine, vol. 285, December
         2, pp. 1288-1292.

Saunders, B.S., "Measuring Community Health Levels," Ameri-
1964   can Journal of Public Health, vol. 54, June, pp.
         1063-1070.

Schaefer, M. and H.E. Hilleboe, "The Health Manpower Crisis,
1967   Cause or Sympton?" American Journal of Public
         Health, vol. 57, January, pp. 6-14.

Scherl, D.J. and J.T. English, "Community Mental Health and
1969   Comprehensive Health Service Programs for the
         Poor," American Journal of Psychiatry, vol. 125,
         June, pp. 1666-1674.

Schonfeld, H.K., et al., "The Development of Standards for
1968   the Audit and Planning of Medical Care," American
         Journal of Public Health, vol. 58, November, pp.
         2097-2110.

Schor, S.S., et al., "An Evaluation of the Periodic Health
    1964   Examination: The Findings in 350 Examinees Who
            Died," Annals of Internal Medicine, vol. 61,
            December, pp. 999-1005.

Schorr, L.B. and J.T. English, "Background, Context and Signi-
    1968   ficant Issues in Neighborhood Health Center Pro-
            grams," Milbank Memorial Fund Quarterly, vol. 46,
            part 1, July, pp. 292-296.

Seago, W.E., "Selecting a Medicare Reimbursement Formula,"
    1968   Journal of Accounting, vol. 126, August, pp.
            31-41.

Sheldon, A., et al., Systems and Medical Care, Cambridge,
    1970   Mass.: MIT Press.

Silver, G.A., Family Medical Care, Cambridge, Mass.: Har-
    1963   vard University Press.

The Size and Shape of the Medical Care Dollar, Chart Book,
    1970   1969, U.S. Department of Health, Education, and
            Welfare, Washington, D.C.:Government Pringing
            Office.

Smalley, H.E., "Management Systems Projects," Hospital
    1967   Management, vol. 103, January, pp. 39-49.

Smallwood, R.D., et al., "A Medical Service Requirements
    1969   Model for Health Systems Design," Proceedings
            of the IEEE, vol. 57, November, pp. 1880-1887.

Smith, H.L., "Two Lines of Authority are One Too Many,"
    1955   Modern Hospital, vol. 84, March, pp. 59-64.

Socioeconomic Issues of Health, Reference Data on, 1971 Re-
    1971   vised Edition, Chicago, Ill.: American Medical
            Association.

Somers, H.M. and A.R. Somers, Doctors, Patients, and Health
    1961   Insurance, Washington, D.C.: The Brookings
            Institute.

Stewart, W.H., "Community Medicine: An American Concept of
1963   Comprehensive Care," Public Health Reports,
        vol. 78, February, pp. 92-100.

Stone, J. M., "National Compulsory Health Insurance: Time
1969   for a Positive Program," Hospitals, vol. 43,
        May 1, pp. 58-63.

Strickland, S.P., "Integration of Medical Research and
1971   Health Policies," Science, vol. 173, September,
        pp. 1093-1103.

Sullivan, D.F., Conceptual Problems in Developing an Index
1966   of Health, Series 2, No. 17, Washington, D.C.:
        U.S. National Center for Health Statistics.

Terris M., "A Social Policy for Health," American Journal
1968   of Public Health, vol. 58, January,p. 1.

Thompson, J.D. and R.B. Fetter, "The Economics of the Mater-
1963   nity Service," Yale Journal of Biology and Medi-
        cine, vol. 36, August, pp. 91-103.

Toffler, A., Future Shock, N.Y.: Random House.
1970

Truxal, J.G., "Technology and Health Services," Proceedings
1969   of the IEEE, vol. 57, November, pp. 1802-1806.

Senate, U.S., Federal Role in Health, Report of the Committee
1970   onGovernment Operations, April 30, Washington,
        D.C.: U.S. Government Printing Office.

Van Brunt, E.E., et al., "A Pilot Data System for a Medical
1969   Center," Proceedings of the IEEE, vol. 57,
        November, pp. 1934-1940.

Vickers, Sir G., "What Sets the Goals of Public Health?"
1958   The Lancet, March 22, pp. 599-604.

Wall Street Journal, "The AMA View of Health Insurance,"
1971   June 8.

Wasyluka, R.G., "New Blood for Tired Hospitals," Harvard
1970   Business Review, vol. 48, Sept.-Oct., pp. 65-74.

Weil, T.P., et al., "Coordinating Health and Management Know-
    1967   ledge for the Training of Health Managers,"
            Journal of Medical Education, vol. 42, August,
            pp. 759-764.

Weinerman, E.R., et al., "Yale Studies in Ambulatory Medical
    1966   Care vs. Determinants of Use of Hospital Emergency
            Services," American Journal of Public Health,
            vol. 56, July, pp. 1037-1056.

Weisbrod, B.A., "Anticipating the Health Needs of Americans:
    1961   Some Economic Projections," Annals of the Ameri-
            can Academy of Political and Social Sciences,
            vol. 337, September, pp. 137-145.

Weisbrod, B.A., Economics of Public Health, Philadelphia,
    1961   Pa.: University of Pennsylvania Press.

Weisbrod, B.A. and R. Fiesler, "Hospitalization Insurance
    1961   and Hospital Utilization," The American Economic
            Review, vol. 51, March, pp. 126-132.

White, K.L., "The Medical School and the Community," Yale
    1967   Journal of Biology and Medicine, vol. 39, June,
            pp. 383-394.

White, K.L., "Research in Medical Care and Health Services
    1968   Systems," Medical Care, vol. 6, March-April,
            pp. 95-100.

White, K.L., "Personal Health Systems Desiderata," Journal
    1971   of the American Medical Association, vol. 218,
            December 13, pp. 1683-1689.

Whittico, J.M., Jr., "Scientific and Social Influences on
    1969   Modern Medical Care Delivery," Proceedings of
            the IEEE, vol. 57, November, pp. 1819-1822.

Wilson, R.N., "The Social Structure of a General Hospital,"
    1963   Annals of the American Academy of Political and
            Social Sciences, vol. 346, March, pp. 67-76.

Part 2.

SYSTEMS

Allen, A.D., Jr., "Systems View of Labor Negotiations,"
    1971   Personnel Journal, vol. 50, February, pp. 103-114.

American Management Association, Organizing for Effective
    1956   Systems Planning and Control, N.Y.: American
            Management Association Press.

Anshen, M., "The Management of Ideas," Harvard Business
    1960   Review, vol. 38, July-August, pp. 99-107.

Arnoff, E.L., "Operations Research and Decision Orientated
    1970   Management Information Systems," Management Ac-
            counting, vol. 51, June, pp. 11-16.

Astrachan, B.M., "Systems Approach to Day Hospitalization,"
    1971   Psychiatric Therapies, vol. 11, pp. 175-182.

Awad, E.M., "Dilemma of the Systems Analyst," Computers
    1970   and Automation, vol. 19, August, pp. 34-38.

Baker, F., and G. O'Brien, "Intersystems Relations and Co-
    1971   ordination of Human Service," American Journal
            of Public Health, vol. 61, January, pp. 130-137.

Battersby, A., Network Analysis for Planning and Scheduling,
    1964   N.Y.: St. Martin's Press.

Berkwitt, G.J., "Systems: Too Much Too Soon?" Dun's Re-
    1968   view, vol. 91, June, pp. 40-42.

Block, A.C., et al., "Manager's Guide to Systems Analysis,"
    1967   Management Review, vol. 56, December, pp. 4-14.

Block, G., "Systems Analysis in Government Operations,"
    1967   Management Science, vol. 14, October, pp. B 41 -
            B 58.

Bloedorn, J.C., "Application of the Systems Analysis Ap-
1970   proach.to Social Welfare Problems and Organization," Public Welfare, vol. 28, July, pp. 280-
284.

Blumberg, M.S., "Medical Manpower-Continuing Crises:
1967   Systems Analysis and Health Manpower," Journal
of the American Medical Association, vol. 201,
September 11, pp. 856-857.

Boguslaw, R., The New Utopians: A Study of System Design
1965   and Social Change, Englewood Cliffs, N.J.:
Prentice-Hall.

Brookfield, K.L., "Role of the Systems Man in Study Teams,"
1970   Journal of Systems Management, vol. 21, October,
pp. 13-15.

Brown, R.A., "Systems Approach to Inventory Management,"
1969   Management Review, vol. 58, March, pp. 27-31.

Brown, W.B., "Systems, Boundaries, and Information Flow,"
1966   Academy of Management Journal, vol. 9, December,
pp. 318-327.

Buckley, W.F., Sociology and Modern Systems Theory, Engle-
1967   wood Cliffs,N.J.: Prentice-Hall.

Burgess, J.H., "Ego Involvement in the Systems Design Pro-
1970   cess," Human Factors, vol. 12, February, pp.
7-12.

Carpenter, H.M., "A System for Storage and Retrieval of
1962   Data from Autopsies," American Journal of
Clinical Pathology, vol. 38, November, pp. 449-
467.

Caruth, D.L., "How Will Total Systems Affect the Corpora-
1969   tion?" Journal of System Management, vol. 20,
February, pp. 10-13.

Chorafas, D.N., Systems and Simulation, N.Y.: Academic
1965   Press.

Cowan, P., "Hospital Systems and Systems of Hospitals,"
1967   Joint Unit for Planning Research, London, England.

Davidson, H.J., "Systems Planning: Art of Corporate Navi-
1967   gation," Financial Executive, vol. 35, April,
          pp. 42-50.

Delon, G.L., and H.E. Smalley, "Systems Approach to Costing
1969   in the Blood Bank," Health Services Research,
          vol. 4, Spring, pp. 53-62.

De Masi, R.J., An Introduction to Business Systems Analysis,
1969   Philippines: Addison-Wesley.

Dror, Y., "Systems Analysis and National Modernization De-
1970   cisions," Academy of Management Journal, vol.
          13, June, pp. 139-152.

Dunn, R.G., and J.T. Howell, "Medical Management Support
1971   Systems," Hospital Progress, vol. 52, September,
          pp. 44-51.

Durbin, R.L., and W.H. Springhall, "Systems Organization
1967   for a Hospital," Hospital Management, vol. 104,
          September, pp. 36-39; October, pp. 57-60; Novem-
          ber, pp. 38-40.

Ehrle, R.A., "Implications of a Systems Approach to Organi-
1965   zation and Management," Personnel Journal, vol.
          44, February, pp. 76-79.

Estafen, B.D., "Methods for Management Research in the
1971   1970's: An Ecological Systems Approach," Aca-
          demy of Management Journal, vol. 14, March, pp.
          51-64.

Feigenbaum, D.S., "Engineering and Management of an Effec-
1968   tive System," Management Science, vol. 14, Aug-
          ust, pp. B 721 - B 732.

Feldman, C.P., "Health Care as a System Problem," Health
1967   Services Research, vol. 2, Summer, pp. 118-120.

Fetter, R.B., and J.D. Thompson, "The Simulation of Hospi-
1965   tal Systems," Operations Research, vol. 13,
          September-October, pp. 689-711.

Finch, J., "Systems Analysis: A Logical Approach to Pro-
1969   fessional Nursing Care," Nursing Forum, vol. 8,
        November 2, pp. 176-190.

Fine, S.A., "Systems Approach to Manpower Development in
1970   Human Services," Public Welfare, vol. 28, Janu-
        ary, pp. 91-97.

Flagle, C.D. (ed.), Operations Research and Systems Engin-
1960   eering, Baltimore, Md.:   Johns Hopkins Press.

Flagle, C.D., "Automated Multiphasic Health Testing and
1971   Services: Total Systems Analysis and Design,"
        Methods of Information in Medicine, vol. 10,
        October, pp. 201-206.

Freeman, J.R., "System Engineering," Hospitals, vol. 44,
1970   April 1, pp. 151-154.

Gagne, R.M., Psychological Principles in Systems Develop-
1962   ment, N.Y.: Holt, Rinehart & Winston.

Gargiulo, G.R., "Network Techniques: A Means for Evalua-
1964   ting Existing Systems and Procedures," Systems
        and Procedures Journal, vol. 15, November,
        pp. 18-25.

Goodman, R.A., "System Diagram of the Functions of a Mana-
1968   ger," California Management Review, vol. 10,
        Summer, pp. 27-38.

Griffin, V.E., "Systems Work Below the Corporate Level,"
1967   Management Accounting, vol. 48, April, pp. 14-20.

Gross, B.M., "Social Systems Accounting," in R.A. Bauer
1967   (ed.) Social Indicators, Cambridge, Mass.: MIT
        Press, pp. 154-271.

Gruber, W.A., "Behavioral Science, Systems Analysis, and
1967   the Failure of Top Management," Industrial
        Management Review, vol. 9, Fall, pp. 37-48.

Hamachek, D.D., "Systems Analysis Precedes Reasons for Con-
1971   sidering a Computer," Hospital Accounting, vol.
        21, January, pp. 24-26.

Hazzard, M.E., "Overview of Systems Theory," Nursing Clinics
1971   of North America, vol. 6, September, pp. 385-393.

Herron, D.P., "Systems Engineering Approach," Automation,
1967   vol. 14, July, pp. 65-70.

Hicks, R.L., "Developing the Top Management Group in a
1971   Total Systems Organization," Personnel Journal,
        vol. 50, September, pp. 675-682.

Hodges, L.C., "Systems and Nursing Care of the Cardiac Sur-
1971   gical Patient," Nursing Clinics of North America,
        vol. 6, September, pp. 415-424.

Hoff, W., "Resolving the Health Manpower Crisis - A Systems
1971   Approach to Utilizing Personnel," American Jour-
        nal of Public Health, vol. 61, December, pp.
        2491-2504.

Holmlund, B.A., "Systems Study of a University Hospital,"
1967   Canadian Medical Association Journal, vol. 97,
        September 16, pp. 746-749.

Howland, D., "A Hospital System Model," Nursing Research,
1963   vol. 12, Fall, pp. 232-236.

Howland, D., "Approaches to the Systems Problem," Nursing
1963   Research, vol. 12, Summer, pp. 172-174.

Hutcheson, B.R., and E.A. Krause, "Systems Analysis and Men-
1969   tal Health Services," Community Mental Health
        Journal, vol. 5, February, pp. 29-45.

IBM Corporation, Hospital Information Systems, Booklet
1963   520-1790, White Plains, N.Y.: IBM, Data Pro-
        cessing Division.

Jarret, I.M., "Key Factor Analysis: The Logic that Relates
1971   the Hospital to Society," Hospital Financial Man-
        agement, vol. 25, April, pp. 4-7.

Jenkins, G.M., and P.V. Youle, "Systems Approach to Manage-
1968   ment," Operations Research, vol. 19, April,
        pp. 5-21.

Kast, F.E., and J.E. Rosenzweig, "System Concepts: Pervas-
1967   iveness and Potential," Management International
        Review, vol. 7, no. 4-5, pp. 87-110.

Kast, F.E., "Dynamic Planning Model: An Application of
1968   Systems Management to Industry," Business Hori-
        zons, vol. 11, June, pp. 61-68.

Katz, J.H., "Simulation of Outpatient Appointment Systems,"
1969   Communications of the A.C.M., vol. 12, April,
        pp. 215-222.

King, W.R., "Systems Concept in Management," Journal of
1967   Industrial Engineering, vol. 18, May, pp. 320-323.

Kovalicik, E.J., "Understanding Systems Engineering," Jour-
1970   nal of Systems Management, vol. 21, September,
        pp. 15-21.

Kraemer, K.I., The Systems Approach in Urban Administration-
1968   Planning Management and Operations, Monticello,
        Ill.: Council of Planning Librarians.

Krueger, R.W., "Systems Analysis, Computers, and the Future
1968   of Professional Services," Computers and Auto-
        mation, vol. 17, July, pp. 34-36.

Lazzaro, N. (ed.), Systems and Procedures: A Handbook for
1968   Business and Industry, 2nd edition, Englewood
        Cliffs, N.J.: Prentice Hall.

Linder, F.E., "Methods for Measuring Population Change. A
1969   Systems Analysis Summary," Vital Health Statis-
        tics, vol. 2, March, pp. 1-18.

McDonough, A.M., Information Economics and Management Sys-
1963   tems, N.Y.: McGraw-Hill.

Mehler, W.R., "A Systems Approach to Managing by Objectives"
1965   Systems and Procedures Journal, vol. 16, Septem-
        ber-October, pp. 12-19.

Miller, E.J., and A.K. Rice, Systems of Organization: The
1967   Control of Task and Sentient Boundaries, N.Y.:
        Barnes & Noble.

Miller, J.G., "Living Systems: Basic Concepts," Behavior-
1965   al Science, vol. 10, July, pp. 193-237.

Morris, R.C., A Study of Hospital Reservation Systems,
1970   Chicago, Ill.: Illinois Institute of Technology.

Morse, F.B., "Private Responsibility for Public Management
1967   (Systems Management Approach)," Harvard Business
        Review, vol. 45, March, pp. 6-21, 178.

Morse, P.M., and L.W. Bacon, Operations Research for Public
1967   Systems, Cambridge, Mass.: M.I.T. Press.

Nadler, G., "Hospital Management Systems are Different,"
1965   Hospital Management, vol. 100, July, pp. 43-45;
        August, pp. 48-51; September, pp. 49-52; Octo-
        ber, pp. 100-106.

Navarro, V., "A Systems Approach to Health Planning,"
1969   Health Services Research, vol. 4, Summer, pp.
        96-111.

Optner, S.L., Systems Analysis for Business and Industrial
1965   Problem Solving, Englewood Cliffs, N.J.:
        Prentice-Hall.

Optner, S.L., Systems Analysis for Business Management,
1968   Englewood Cliffs, N.J.: Prentice-Hall.

Palumbo, D.J., et al., "A Systems Analysis of Local Public
1969   Health Departments," American Journal of Public
        Health, vol. 59, April, pp. 673-679.

Pounds, W.F., "Nature of Systems," Conference Board Record,
1970   vol. 7, August, pp. 49-51.

Quade, E.S., "Systems Analysis Techniques for Planning,
1966   Programming, Budgeting," The RAND Corp., No.
        3322, March.

Ramo, S., Cure for Chaos: Fresh Solution to Social Prob-
1969   lems Through the Systems Approach, N.Y.: David
        McKay Co.

Randall, C.B., <u>Systems and Procedures for Business Data</u>
1968   <u>Processing</u>, Cincinnati, Ohio: South-Western
Publishing Co.

Rapoport, A., "Modern Systems Theory--An Outlook for
1970   Coping with Change," <u>General Systems</u>, vol.
15, pp. 15-25.

Schaeffer, R.G., "Systems in Managing Change," <u>Conference</u>
1970   <u>Board Record</u>, vol. 7, August, pp. 48-49.

Schlesinger, J.R., <u>Systems Analysis and the Political Pro-</u>
1967   <u>cess</u>, Santa Monica, Calif.: The RAND Corp.

Schoderbek, P.P., <u>Management Systems</u>, N.Y.: John Wiley &
1967   Sons.

Schumaker, C.J., Jr., "Systems Management Study: A Train-
1971   ing Tool for an Administrative Residency Program,"
<u>Hospital Progress</u>, vol. 52, August, pp. 58ff.

Seiler, J.A., <u>Systems Analysis in Organizational Behavior</u>,
1967   Homewood, Ill.: Richard D. Irwin.

Sheldon, A., et al., <u>Systems and Medical Care</u>, Cambridge,
1970   Mass.: M.I.T. Press.

Shrode, W.A., and R.E. Wilkinson, "Toward a Systems Model
1970   of Managerial Performance," <u>Journal of Systems</u>
<u>Management</u>, vol. 21, September, pp. 29-33.

Sims, N.H., "Systems Analysis of Pediatrician Efficiency,"
1971   <u>Johns Hopkins Medical Journal</u>, vol. 128, January,
pp. 30-40.

Singh, A.J., <u>Transportation Systems for Maternity and In-</u>
1968   <u>fant Care Project Patients</u>, technical memorandum
No. 140, Cleveland, Ohio: Case Western Reserve
University, Department of Operations Research.

Stone, A.R., "The Interdisciplinary Research Team," <u>Jour-</u>
1969   <u>nal of Applied Behavioral Science,</u> vol. 5, July-
August-September, pp. 351-365.

Stout, W.J., "How the Systems Approach Aids Administrative
    1971   Problem-Solving," Hospital Topics, vol. 49,
            November, pp. 42-48.

Sussams, J.E., "Business Systems Analysis - a New Approach,"
    1968   Operations Research, vol. 19, April, pp. 85-91.

"Systems Analysis Approach to Hospital Design," Architec-
    1970   tural Record, vol. 147, March, pp. 112-115.

"Systems Research in Delivery of Health Services," Health
    1970   Services Research, vol. 5, Spring, pp. 60-61.

"Systems Research for Improving the Delivery of Health
    1971   Care," Health Services Research, vol. 6, Spring,
            pp, 83-85.

Thimm, A.L., "General Systems Theory: A Tool for Social
    1970   Analysis," Journal of Systems Management, vol.
            21, October, pp. 16-21.

Thomas, D.S.H., "Management Planning and Control of Systems,"
    1970   Managerial Planning, vol. 19, July-August, pp.
            1-7.
Tilles, S., "Manager's Job: A Systems Approach," Harvard
    1963   Business Review, vol. 41, January, pp. 73-81.

Weinerman, E.R., "Research on Comparative Health Service
    1971   Systems," Medical Care, vol. 9, May-June, pp.
            272-290.

Wilson, I.G., and M.E. Wilson, Information, Computer, and
    1965   Systems Design, N.Y.: John Wiley & Sons.

Wilson, R., "Systems Analysis in Health Sciences Educational
    1969   Planning," Canadian Medical Journal, vol. 100,
            April 19, pp. 715-723.

Yerby, A., "Health Care Systems, Some International Com-
    1970   parisons," Technological Review, vol. 72, April,
            pp. 25-27.

Young, S., Management: A System Analysis, Glenview, Ill.:
    1966   Scott, Foresman and Co.

Zaino, L.F., "Defense Plans Hospital Systems Design,"
  1969   Engineering News-Record, vol. 18, February 6,
          p. 84.

Zolber, K., "Food Service: Research on Assembly-Serve
  1971   Systems," Hospitals, vol. 45, January 16, pp.
          83-87.

Part 3.

ORGANIZATIONS

Akers, R.L., "Framework for the Comparative Study of Group
1970   Cohesion: The Professions," _Pacific Sociological Review_, vol. 13, April, pp. 73-85.

Akers, R.L., and R. Quinney, "Differential Organization of
1968   Health Professions: A Comparative Analysis,"
American Sociological Review, vol. 33, February,
pp. 104-121.

Allen, E.M., "The Manager in the Middle: Coping with Pres-
1970   sure from Both Sides," _Management Review_, vol.
59, November, pp. 41-45.

Argyris, C., _Understanding Organizational Behavior_, Homewood,
1960   Ill.: Dorsey Press.

Argyris, C., _Interpersonal Competence and Organizational_
1962   _Effectiveness_, Homewood, Ill.: Richard D. Irwin.

Argyris, C., _Integrating the Individual and the Organiza-_
1964   _tion_, N.Y.: John Wiley & Sons.

Argyris, C., _Organization and Innovation_, Homewood, Ill.:
1965   Richard D. Irwin.

Athos, A., and R.F. Coffey, _Behavior in Organization: A_
1968   _Multidimensional View_, Englewood Cliffs, N.J.:
Prentice-Hall.

Barnard, C.I., _The Functions of the Executive_, Cambridge,
1966   Mass.: Harvard University Press.

Barnes, L.B., _Organizational Systems and Engineering_
1960   _Groups: A Comparative Study of Two Technical_
Systems in Industry, Boston: Division of Research, Harvard Business School, Harvard University.

Bass, B.M., _Organizational Psychology_, Boston: Allyn &
1965   Bacon.

_29_

Bauer, R.A. (ed.), <u>Social Indicators</u>, Cambridge, Mass.:
1966   M.I.T. Press.

Bauer, R.A., "Social Feedback," <u>The Annals of the American</u>
1967   <u>Academy of Political and Social Science</u>, vol.
373, September, pp. 180-192.

Bauerschmidt, A.D., "Hospital as a Prototype Organization,"
1970   <u>Hospital Administration</u>, vol. 15, Spring, pp.
6-14.

Beckhard, R., <u>Organizational Development: Strategies and</u>
1969   <u>Models</u>, Reading, Mass.: Addison-Wesley.

Bennis, W.G., <u>The Planning of Change</u>, N.Y.: Holt, Rinehart
1961   & Winston.

Bennis, W.G., "A New Role for the Behavioral Sciences:
1963   Effecting Organizational Change," <u>Administra-</u>
<u>tive Science Quarterly</u>, vol. 8, September, pp.
125-165.

Bennis, W.G., <u>Changing Organizations</u>, N.Y.: McGraw-Hill.
1966

Blake, R.R., et al., "Breakthrough in Organization Develop-
1964   ment," <u>Harvard Business Review</u>, vol. 42, November, pp. 133-135.

Blau, P.M., and R.W. Scott, <u>Formal Organization: A Compara-</u>
1962   <u>tive Approach</u>, San Francisco, Calif.: Chandler
Publishing Co.

Boguslaw, R., <u>The New Utopians</u>, Englewood Cliffs, N.J.:
1965   Prentice-Hall.

Boulding, E., et al., <u>Conflict Management in Organization</u>,
1961   Ann Arbor, Michigan: Foundation for Research on
Human Behavior, University of Michigan.

Bower, R. (ed.), <u>Research Conference on Behavior in Organi-</u>
1966   <u>zations</u>, A research symposium. Athens, Ga.:
University of Georgia Press.

Braudy, R.A., Organization: Automation and Society. The
1961   Scientific Revolution in Industry, Berkeley,
        Calif.: University of California Press.

Brown, B.J.R., Teaching Hospital Organizational Identity
1970   and Climate Inventory, Milwaukee, Wisc.:
        Marquette University Press.

Brown, C.C., "Pattern of Management for the Seventies,"
1970   Columbia Journal of World Business, vol. 5,
        November, pp. 23-29.

Burke, W.W., "Comparison of Management Development and Or-
1971   ganization Development," Journal of Applied
        Behavioral Sciences, vol. 7, September-October,
        pp. 569-579.

Burns, T., and G.M. Stalker, The Management of Innovation,
1961   London: Tavistock Publications.

Carpenter, W.H., Corporate Organization in Non-Profit Non-
1971   governmental Short-Term General Hospitals in
        the United States, Birmingham, Ala.: The Univer-
        sity of Alabama Press.

Clark, J.V., "Motivation in Work Groups: A Tentative View,"
1960-61 Human Organizations, vol. 19, Winter, pp. 199-208.

Cohen, A.M., et al., "Experiments in Organizational Embed-
1969   dedness," Administrative Science Quarterly, vol.
        14, June, pp. 208-221.
Cooper, W.W., et al., New Perspectives in Organization
1964   Research, N.Y.: John Wiley & Sons.

Crockett, W.J., "Team Building--One Approach to Organiza-
1970   tional Development," Journal of Applied Be-
        havioral Science, vol. 6, pp. 291-306.

Crozier, M., The Bureaucratic Phenomenon, Chicago: Univer-
1964   sity of Chicago Press.

Dalton, G.W., and P.R. Lawrence with J. Lorsch, Organiza-
1970   tional Structure and Design, Homewood, Ill.:
        Richard D. Irwin.

Davis, K., <u>Human Relations at Work</u>, N.Y.: McGraw-Hill.
  1967

DeMaagd, G.P., "Matrix Management," <u>Datamation</u>, vol. 16,
  1970   October 15, pp. 46-49.

DeNeufville, R., "Systems Analysis - A Decision Process,"
  1970   <u>Industrial Management Review</u>, vol. 11, Spring,
          pp. 49-58.

DeSpelder, B., "Designing the Participative Decision-
  1964   Making System," <u>Systems and Procedures Journal</u>,
          vol. 15, January, pp. 20-24.

Drucker, P., <u>The Effective Executive</u>, N.Y.: Harper & Row.
  1967

Emery, F.E., and E.L. Trist, "The Causal Texture of Organi-
  1965   zational Environments," <u>Human Relations</u>, vol.
          18, pp. 21-32.

Etzioni, A., "Two Approaches to Organizational Analysis:
  1960   A Critique and a Suggestion," <u>Administrative
          Science Quarterly</u>, vol. 5, September, pp. 257-278.

Etzioni, A., <u>A Comparative Analysis of Complex Organiza-
  1961   tions</u>, N.Y.: Free Press.

Etzioni, A.,<u>Complex Organizations, a Sociological Reader</u>,
  1961   N.Y.: Holt, Rinehart & Winston.

Etzioni, A., <u>A Modern Organization</u>, Englewood Cliffs, N.J.:
  1964   Prentice-Hall.

Evan, W.M., "Indices of Hierarchical Structure of Industrial
  1963   Organizations," <u>Management Science</u>, vol. 9,
          April, pp. 468-477.

Evans, M.C., "Leadership and Motivation: A Core Concept,"
  1970   <u>Academy of Management Journal</u>, vol. 13, March,
          pp. 91-102.

Fink, S.L., J. Beak, and K. Taddeo, "Organizational Crisis
  1971   and Change," <u>Journal of Applied Behavioral
          Science</u>, vol. 7, pp. 15-37.

Flagle, C.D., "The Problem of Organization for Hospital In-
1960   patient Care," in M. Verhulst, (ed.),Management
        Sciences: Models and Techniques, vol. 11, New
        York: Pergamon Press. pp. 275-287.

Freidson, E., and J.H. Mann, "Organizational Dimensions of
1971   Large-Scale Group Medical Practice," American
        Journal of Public Health, vol. 61, April, pp.
        786-795.

Gellerman, S., "Behavioral Strategies," California Manage-
1969   ment Review, vol. 12, Winter, pp. 45-51.

Georgopoulos, B.S., "Hospital Organization and Administra-
1964   tion, Prospects and Perspectives," Hospital
        Administration, vol. 9, no. 3, pp. 23-35.

Georgopoulos, B.S., "Normative Structure Variables and Or-
1965   ganizational Behavior: A Comparative Study,"
        Human Relations, vol. 18, pp. 155-169.

Golembiewski, R.T., and F.K. Gibson, (eds.), Managerial
1967   Behavior and Organization Demands: Management as
        a Linking of Levels of Interaction, Chicago,
        Ill.: Rand McNally.

Guest, R.H., Organizational Change. The Effect of Success-
1962   ful Leadership, Homewood, Ill.: Richard D.Irwin.

Hage, J., and M. Aiken, "Program Change and Organizational
1967   Properties--A Comparative Analysis," American
        Journal of Sociology, vol. 72, March, pp. 503-
        519.

Haire, M., E. Ghiselli, and L. Porter, Managerial Thinking,
1966   N.Y.: John Wiley & Sons.

Harrison, R., "Choosing the Depth of Organizational Inter-
1970   vention," Journal of Applied Behavioral Science,
        vol. 6, no. 2, pp. 181-202.

Harvey, E., "Technology and the Structure of Organizations,"
1968   American Sociological Review, vol. 33, April,
        pp. 247-259.

Hicks, H.G., The Management of Organizations, N.Y.:
1967   McGraw-Hill.

Hirschman, A.O., Exit, Voice and Loyalty: Response to De-
1970   cline in Firms, Organizations and States,
        Cambridge, Mass.: Harvard University Press.

Hodge, B.J., Management and Organizational Behavior,
1970   N.Y.: John Wiley & Sons.

Homans, G.C., Social Behavior: Its Elementary Forms,
1961   N.Y.: Harcourt, Brace and World.

House, R.J., "Role Conflict and Multiple Authority in Com-
1970   plex Organization," California Management Review,
        vol. 12, Summer, pp. 53-60.

Hunt, J.G., and J.W. Hill, "The New Look in Motivation
1969   Theory for Organizational Research," Human
        Organization, vol. 28, Summer, pp. 100-109.

Hunt, R., "Technology and Organization," Academy of Manage-
1970   ment Journal, vol. 13, September, pp. 235-252.

Hutchinson, J.G., Organizations, Theory and Classical Con-
1967   cepts, N.Y.: Holt, Rinehart & Winston.

Inkson, J.H.K., D.J. Pugh, and D.J. Hickson, "Organization
1970   Context and Structure. An Abbreviated Replica-
        tion," Academy of Management Journal, vol. 13,
        September, pp. 318-329.

Ivancevich, J.M., "Analysis of Control Bases and of Control
1970   Satisfaction in an Organizational Setting,"
        Academy of Management Journal, vol. 13, December,
        pp. 427-436.

Jenks, R.S., "An Action-Research Approach to Organizational
1970   Change," Journal of Applied Behavioral Science,
        vol. 6, no. 2, pp. 131-149.

Jones, G.N., "Strategies and Tactics of Planned Organizat-
1965   ional Change: Case Examples in the Modernization
        Process of Traditional Societies," Human Organi-
        zation, vol. 24, Fall, pp. 192-200.

Kahn, R., et al., Organizational Stress, Studies in Role
1964   Conflict and Ambiguity, N.Y.: John Wiley & Sons.

Kahn, R., and E. Boulding, Power and Conflict in Organiza-
1964   tions, N.Y.: Basic Books.

Kast, F., and J. Rosenzweig, Organization and Management:
1969   A Systems Approach, N.Y.: McGraw-Hill.

Katz, D., and B.S. Georgopoulos, "Organizations in a
1971   Changing World," Journal of Applied Behavioral
        Science, vol. 7, May-June, pp. 342-370.

Katz, D., and R.L. Kahn, The Social Psychology of Organi-
1966   zations, N.Y.: John Wiley & Sons, pp. 9 and 13.

Katz, R.L., and J.A. Seiler, Management Behavior: The
1962   Psychology of Organization, Boston: Division of
        Research, Harvard Business School.

Kaufman, H., and D. Seidman, "The Morphology of Organiza-
1970   tion," Administrative Science Quarterly, vol.
        15, December, pp. 439-451.

Kelly, J., Organization Behavior, Homewood, Ill.: Richard
1969   D. Irwin.

Klatzky, S.R., "Relationship of Organization Size to Com-
1970   plexity and Coordination," Administrative
        Science Quarterly, vol. 15, December, pp. 438-448.

Krupp, S., Patterns in Organization Analysis, N.Y.: Holt,
1964   Rinehart & Winston.

Kuethe, J.L.,and B. Levensen, "Conceptions of Organizational
1964   Worth," American Journal of Sociology, vol. 70,
        November, pp. 342-348.

Lammers, C.J., "Power and Participation in Decision Making
1967   in Formal Organizations," American Journal of
        Sociology, vol. 73, no. 2, pp. 201-216.

Lawrence, P.R., The Changing of Organizational Behavior
1958   Patterns: A Case Study of Decentralization,
        Boston: Division of Research, Harvard Business
        School, see Chapter X.

Lawrence, P.R., <u>Organizational Behavior and Administration:</u>
    1961   <u>Cases, Concepts and Research Findings</u>, Homewood,
            Ill.: Dorsey Press, pp. 126-167.

Learned, E.P.,and A.T. Sproat, <u>Organization Theory and</u>
    1966   <u>Policy, Notes for Analysis</u>, Homewood, Ill.:
            Richard D. Irwin.

Leibenstein, H., <u>Economic Theory and Organizational Analysis</u>,
    1960   N.Y.: Harper & Row.

Levine, S., and P.E. White, "Exchange as a Conceptual
    1961   Framework for Study of Interorganizational Relat-
            ionships," <u>Administrative Science Quarterly,</u> vol.
            5, March, pp. 583-601.

Likert, R., <u>The Human Organization: Its Management and</u>
    1967   <u>Value</u>, N.Y.: McGraw-Hill.

Linton, C.B., <u>Analysis of Organizational Structures in</u>
    1970   <u>Hospital-Based Extended Care Facilities</u>,
            Chicago, Ill.: American College of Hospital
            Administrators.

Lippit, G.L., <u>Organizational Renewal, Achieving Viability</u>
    1969   <u>in a Changing World</u>, N.Y.: Appleton-Century-
            Crofts.

Litterer, J.A., <u>The Analysis of Organizations</u>, N.Y.: John
    1965   Wiley & Sons.

Lupton, T., <u>Management and the Social Sciences</u>, London:
    1966   Hutchinson.

MacGregor, D.M., <u>The Human Side of Enterprise</u>, Cambridge,
    1960   Mass.: M.I.T. Press. New York: McGraw-Hill.

Mailick, S. (ed.), <u>Concepts and Issues in Administrative</u>
    1962   <u>Behavior</u>, Englewood Cliffs, N.J.: Prentice-Hall.

March, J., <u>Handbook of Organizations</u>, Chicago, Ill.: Rand
    1965   McNally & Co.

McFeely, W.M., "Multilayered Management: A Three-Ply
  1971   Concept of Organization Offers a New Model for
          Effecting Change," Conference Board Record,
          vol. 8, March, pp. 25-29.

Mee, J.F., "Profile of the Future: Speculation About Human
  1971   Organization in the 21st Century," Business Hori-
          zons, vol. 14, February, pp. 5-16.

Miller, E.J., Systems of Organization. The Control of
  1967   Task and Sentient Boundary, London: Tavistock
          Publications.

Mohr, L.B., "Organizational Technology and Organizational
  1971   Structure: 13 Local Health Departments," Admini-
          strative Science Quarterly, vol. 16, December,
          pp. 444-459.

Morse, J.J., and J.W. Lorsch, "Beyond Theory: An Effective
  1970   Organization Must be Designated to Fit its Task
          and its People," Harvard Business Review, vol.
          48, May, pp. 61-68.

Murray, J.A., "A Sociometric Approach to Organizational
  1970   Analysis," California Management Review, vol. 13,
          Fall, pp. 59-67.

Newman, A.D., and R.W. Rowbottom, Organization Analysis.
  1968   A Guide to Better Understanding of Structural
          Problems, Carbondale, Ill.: Southern Illinois
          University Press.

Newman, W.H., Administrative Actions--The Techniques of
  1963   Organization and Management, second edition,
          Englewood Cliffs, N.J.: Prentice-Hall.

O'Brien, G.E., "Leadership in Organizational Settings,"
  1969   Journal of Applied Behavioral Science, vol. 5,
          no. 1, pp. 45-61.

Odiorne, G.S., Management by Objectives: A System for
  1965   Management Leadership, N.Y.: Pitman Publishing
          Corp.

Perrow, C.A., "A Framework for the Comparative Analysis of
1967   Organizations," <u>American Sociological Review</u>,
         vol. 32, pp. 194-208.

Pondy, L.R., "Effect of Size, Complexity and Ownership on
1969   Administrative Intensity," <u>Administrative Science</u>
         <u>Quarterly</u>, vol. 14, March, pp. 47-60.

Poppel, H.L., "Matrix Organization Designs," <u>Business Hori-</u>
1961   <u>zons</u>, vol. 14, February, pp. 29-40.

Porter, L.W., and E.E. Lawler, III, "Properties of Organi-
1965   zational Structure in Relation to Job Attitudes
         and Job Behavior," <u>Psychological Bulletin</u>, vol.
         64, no. 1, pp. 23-51.

Porter, L.W., and E.E. Lawler, III, "The Effects of 'tall'
1964   versus 'flat' Organization Structures on Mana-
         gerial Job Satisfaction," <u>Personnel Psychology</u>,
         vol. 17, no. 2, pp. 135-148.
Presthus, R., <u>The Organizational Society: An Analysis and</u>
1962   <u>a Theory</u>, N.Y.: Vintage Books (Knopf).

Pugh, D.S., et al., "A Conceptual Scheme for Organizational
1963   Analysis," <u>Administrative Science Quarterly</u>,
         vol. 8, December, pp. 289-315.

Pugh, D.S., D.J. Hickson, and C.R. Hinings, <u>Writers on</u>
1964   <u>Organizations</u>, London: Hutchinson.

Randall, L.K., "Common Questions and Tentative Answers
1971   Regarding Organization Development," <u>California</u>
         <u>Management Review</u>, vol. 13, Spring, pp. 45-52.

Reddin, W.J., "Managing Organizational Change," <u>Hospital</u>
1970   <u>Administration</u>, vol. 15, Winter, pp. 79-86.

Revans, R.W., "The Hospital as an Organization--A Study in
1960   Communication and Morale," in M. Verhulst (ed.),
         <u>Management Sciences Models and Techniques</u>, vol.
         11, N.Y.: Pergamon Press, pp. 17-24.

Rice, A.K., "Individual, Group, and Inter-group Processes,"
1969   <u>Human Relations</u>, vol. 22, December, pp. 565-584.

Rizzo, J.R., et al., "Role Conflict and Ambiguity in Complex
1970   Organizations," Administrative Science Quarterly,
        vol. 15, June, pp. 150-163.

Rowbottom, R.W., "Emerging Patterns of Hospital Organiza-
1971   tion," British Hospital Journal and Social Ser-
        vice, May 8, 15, 22 and 29.

Rubinstein, A.H., and J. C. Haberstroh (eds.), Some Theories
1966   of Organization, Homewood, Ill.: Richard D. Irwin.

Samuel,K., and B.F. Mannheim, "A Multidimensional Approach
1970   toward a Typology of Bureaucracy," Administra-
        tive Science Quarterly, vol. 15, June, pp. 216-229.

Schein, E.H., Organizational Psychology, Englewood Cliffs,
1965   N.J.: Prentice-Hall.

Scott, W.G., Organization Theory, A Behavioral Analysis for
1967   Management, Homewood, Ill.: Richard D. Irwin.

Scott, W.R., "Some Implications of Organization Theory for
1966   Research on Health Services," Milbank Memorial
        Fund Quarterly, October, vol. 44, part 2, pp.
        35-59.

Seashore, S. (ed.), Assessing Organization Performance with
1964   Behavioral Measurement, Ann Arbor, Michigan:
        Foundation for Research on Human Behavior.

Simpson, R.L. and W.H. Gulley, "Goals, Environmental Pres-
1962   sures and Organizational Characteristics," Ameri-
        can Sociological Review, vol. 27, June, pp. 344-
        351.
Smith, C.G., "A Comparative Analysis of Some Conditions and
1966   Consequences of Intra-Organizational Conflict,"
        Administrative Science Quarterly, vol. 10, March,
        pp. 504-529.

Taguiri, R., "Value Orientations of Managers and Scientists,"
1964   in C.D. Orth III, et al. (eds.), Administering
        Research and Development, Homewood, Ill.: Richard
        D. Irwin.

Tannenbaum, A.S., <u>Social Psychology of the Work Organization</u>,
1966   Belmont, Calif.: Wadsworth Publishing Co.

Tannenbaum, A.S. (ed.), <u>Control in Organizations</u>, N.Y.:
1968   McGraw-Hill.

Tannenbaum, A.S., and C.G. Smith, "Effects of Member Influ-
1964   ence in an Organization: Phenomenology versus
        Organization Structure," <u>Journal of Abnormal</u>
        <u>and Social Psychology</u>, vol. 69, no. 4, pp. 401-410.

Thompson, J.D. (ed.), <u>Approaches to Organizational Design</u>,
1966   Pittsburgh, Pa.: University of Pittsburgh Press.

Thompson, J.D., <u>Organization in Action. Social Science</u>
1967   <u>Bases for Administrative Theory</u>, N.Y.: McGraw-
        Hill.

Thornton, R., "Organizational Involvement and Commitment
1970   to Organization and Profession," <u>Administrative</u>
        <u>Science Quarterly</u>, vol. 15, December, pp. 417-427.

Tiger, L., <u>Men in Groups</u>, N.Y.: Random House.
1969

Tosi, H., "Organization Stress, A Moderation of the Relation-
1971   ship Influence and Role Response," <u>Academy of</u>
        <u>Management Journal</u>, vol. 14, March, pp. 7ff.

Trist, F.E., et al., <u>Organizational Choice</u>, London: Tavis-
1963   tock Publications.

Wall, H.R., "Reconciling Organization and Personal Goals,"
1970   <u>Personnel Journal</u>, vol. 49, January, pp. 41-44.

Warner, K.W., and S.G. Miller, "Organizational Problems in
1964   Two Types of Voluntary Associations," <u>American</u>
        <u>Journal of Sociology</u>, vol. 69, May, pp. 654-657.

Whitaker, G. (ed.), <u>T-Group Training: Group Dynamics in</u>
1965   <u>Management Education</u>, Oxford: Blackwell.

White, H., <u>Chain of Opportunity. Systems Models of Mobili-</u>
1970   <u>ty in Organizations</u>, Cambridge, Mass.: Harvard
        University Press.

Whyte, W.H.,Jr., The Organization Man, N.Y.: Simon &
    1956   Schuster, Inc.

Wright, R.W., "Organizational Ambiente: Management and
    1971   Environment in Chile," Academy of Management
            Journal, vol. 14, March, pp. 65-74.

Young, S., Management: A Decision-Making Approach,
    1968   Belmont, Calif.: Dickenson Publishing Co.

Zaleznik, A., Human Dilemmas of Leadership, N.Y.: Harper
    1966   & Row.

Zaleznik, A., "Managerial Behavior and Interpersonal Com-
    1967   petence," in W.A. Hill,and D.M. Egan (eds.),
            Readings in Organizational Theory: A Behavioral
            Approach, Boston, Mass.: Allyn & Bacon, Inc.
            pp. 228-241.

Zand, D.E., et al., "The Impact of an Organizational Devel-
    1969   ment Program on Perceptions of Interpersonal,
            Group, and Organization Functioning," Journal
            of Applied Behavioral Science, vol. 5, no. 3,
            pp. 393-410.

Part 4.

STRUCTURAL ASPECTS OF DECISION-MAKING

Ackoff, R.L., Scientific Method: Optimizing Applied Re-
    1962   Research Decisions, N.Y.: John Wiley & Sons.

Aitchison, J., "Decision-Making in Clinical Medicine,"
    1970   Journal of the Royal College of Physicians of
            London, vol. 4, April, pp. 195-202.

Alker, H.A., and M.G. Hermann, "Are Bayesian Decisions
    1971   Artificially Intelligent? The Effect of Task
            and Personality on Conservatism in Processing
            Information," Journal of Personality and Social
            Psychology, vol. 19, July, pp. 31-44 .

Andrews, C.T., Financial and Statistical Reports for Admini-
    1968   strative Decision-Making in Hospitals, Bloomington,
            Indiana: Indiana University Press.

Aoki, M., Optimization of Stochastic Systems, N.Y.:
    1967   Academic Press.

Barish, N., Economic Analysis for Engineering and Managerial
    1962   Decision-Making, N.Y.: McGraw-Hill.

Beer, S., Decision and Control, N.Y.: John Wiley & Sons.
    1966

Blecke, C., Financial Analysis for Decision-Making, Engle-
    1966   wood Cliffs, N.J.: Prentice-Hall.

Boot, J., Mathematical Reasoning in Economics and Manage-
    1967   ment Science, Englewood Cliffs, N.J.: Prentice-
            Hall.

Boot, J., Statistical Analysis for Managerial Decisions,
    1970   Englewood Cliffs, N.J.: Prentice-Hall.

Bork, D., "Decision Theory: An Operations Research Tool,"
    1968   Systems and Procedures Journal, vol. 19, May,
            pp. 24-26.

Boulden, J.B., and E.S. Buffa, "Corporate Models: On Line,
1970   Real Time Systems," Harvard Business Review,
        vol. 48, July, pp. 65-83.

Bracken, J., and R.M. Soland, "Statistical Decision Models
1967   for Brokering," Management Science, vol. 15,
        July, pp. 619-625.

Brady, R.H., "Computers in Top Level Decision-Making,"
1967   Harvard Business Review, vol. 45, July, pp.
        67-76.

Bray, J., "Decision Making in Government," Operational
1968   Research Quarterly, vol. 19, April, pp. 25-35.

Braybrooke, D., and C.E. Lindblom, A Strategy of Decision,
1963   Glencoe, N.Y.: Free Press of Glencoe.

Bross, I.D., Design for Decision, N.Y.: Macmillan.
1953

Campagna, A.S., "Capital Appropriations and the Investment
1968   Decision," Review of Economics and Statistics,
        vol. 50, May, pp. 207-214.

Carson, J.R., "Business Games: A Technique for Teaching
1967   Decision-Making," National Association of
        Accountants Journal, vol. 49, October, pp. 31-35.

Chesebrough, W.C., "Decision Tables as a Systems Technique,"
1970   Computers and Automation, vol. 19, April, pp.
        30-33.

Churchman, C.W., Prediction and Optimal Decision, Engle-
1961   wood Cliffs, N.J.: Prentice-Hall.

Cohen, J., Behaviour in Uncertainty and its Social Impli-
1965   cations, N.Y.: Basic Books.

Davidson, S., et al., Decision-Making, An Experimental Ap-
1957   proach, Stanford, Calif.: Stanford University
        Press.

"Decision Making in Hospitals," pp. 52-54;
"Decision Making in Local Government," pp. 47-51;
"Decision Making in Manpower Planning," pp. 129-132;
"Decision Making in Research and Development," pp. 133-135;
  1968   Operational Research Quarterly, vol. 19, April.

Dickaut, J.W., "Accounting Information in Decision-Making,"
  1969   Management Services, vol. 6, January, pp. 49-55.

Dowling, W.L., "Application of Linear Programming to Decision
  1971   Making in Hospitals," Hospital Administration
          (Chicago), vol. 16, Summer, pp. 66-75.

Dyckman, T.R.,and A.K. McAdams, Management Decision Making
  1969   Under Uncertainty, N.Y.: Macmillan.

Emory, W., Making Management Decisions, Boston: Houghton,
  1968   Mifflin Co.

Fergus, R.M., "Introduction to Decision Tables," Systems
  1968   and Procedures Journal, vol. 19, July, pp. 24-27.

Fishburn, P.C., "Sensitivity of Decisions to Probability
  1968   Estimation Errors: A Re-examination," Operations
          Research, vol. 16, March, pp. 254-267.

Fleming, J.E., "Study of a Business Decision," California
  1966   Management Review, vol. 9, Winter, pp. 51-56.

Ford, C.H., and E.C. Bursk, "Organizing for Faster Decis-
  1971   ions," Management Review, vol. 60, April, pp.
          4-19.

Gentry, J.T., "Planning of Community Health Services:
  1971   Facilitating Rational Decision-Making," Inquiry,
          vol. 8, September, pp. 4-21.

Gillis, F., Managerial Economics, Reading, Mass.: Addison
  1969   Wesley.

Glover, F., "Management Decision and Integer Programming,"
  1969   Accounting Review, vol. 44, April, pp. 300-303.

Grawoig, D.E., Decision Mathematics, N.Y.: McGraw-Hill.
  1967

Grayson, C., Jr., <u>Decisions Under Uncertainty: Drilling</u>
  1960   <u>Decisions by Oil and Gas Operators</u>, Cambridge,
          Mass.: Harvard Business School.

Greenwood, W., <u>Decision Theory and Information Systems</u>,
  1969   Cincinnati, Ohio: South Western Publishing Co.

Hadley, G., <u>Introduction to Probability and Statistical</u>
  1967   <u>Decision Theory</u>, San Francisco, Calif.:
          Holden-Day.

Hague, D.G., <u>Managerial Economics</u>, N.Y.: John Wiley & Sons.
  1969

Hall, J., and M.S. Williams, "Group Dynamics Training and
  1970   Improved Decision-Making," <u>Journal of Applied</u>
          <u>Behavioral Science</u>, vol. 6, January-March,
          pp. 39-68.

Hausman, W.H., "Sequential Decisions Problems: A Model to
  1969   Exploit Existing Forecasters," <u>Management Science</u>
          vol. 16, October, pp. 93-111.

Hein, L.W., <u>The Quantitative Approach to Managerial De-</u>
  1967   <u>cisions</u>, Englewood Cliffs, N.J.: Prentice-Hall.

Hirshleifer, J., "The Bayesian Approach to Statistical De-
  1961   cision: An Exposition," <u>Journal of Business</u>
          <u>of the University of Chicago</u>, vol. 34, June,
          pp. 471-489.

Jackson, J.R., "On Decision Theory Under Competition,"
  1968   <u>Management Science</u>, vol. 15, September, pp. 12-32.

Jedamus, P., and R. Frame, <u>Business Decision Theory</u>, N.Y.:
  1969   McGraw-Hill.

Jones, C.H., "At Last: Real Computer Power for Decision
  1970   Makers," <u>Harvard Business Review</u>, vol. 48,
          September-October, pp. 75-89.

Kaplan, S., and N.N. Barish, "Decision Making Allowing for
  1967   Uncertainty of Future Investment Opportunities,"
          <u>Management Science</u>, vol. 13, June, pp. 569-577.

Kassouf, S.T., Normative Decision Theory, Englewood Cliffs,
1971   N.J.: Prentice-Hall.

Kogan, N., and M.A. Wallach, Risk Taking, N.Y.: Holt,
1964   Rinehart & Winston.

Kunreuther, H., "Extension of Bowman's Theory on Managerial
1969   Decision-Making," Management Science, vol. 15,
        April, pp. 415-439.

Little, J.D.C., "Model and Managers: The Concept of a
1970   Decision Calculus," Management Science, vol. 16,
        April, pp. 466-485.

Lopez, F., Evaluating Executive Decision Making, N.Y.:
1966   American Management Association Press.

Lorei, T.W., and L. Gurel, "A Systematic Approach to Dis-
1971   position of Decisions," American Journal of
        Psychiatry, vol. 128, September, pp. 281-285.

Luckman, J., "Approach to Management of Design," Opera-
1967   tional Research Quarterly, vol. 18, December,
        pp. 345-358.

Lusted, L.B., Introduction to Medical Decision Making,
1968   Springfield, Ill.: Charles C. Thomas.

Magee, J.F., "How to Use Decision Trees in Capital Invest-
1964   ment," Harvard Business Review, vol. 42,
        September-October, pp. 75-95.

Mao, J.C.T., Quantitative Analysis of Financial Decisions,
1969   N.Y.: Macmillan.

McFarlane, D.D., and I. Horowitz, "Risk and the Business
1968   Decision," Harvard Business Review, vol. 46,
        July-August, pp. 81-90.

Meier, A., "Entrepreneural Decision Making and Electronic
1967   Data Processing," Management International Re-
        view, vol. 7, November, pp. 3-24.

Miller, I.M., "Computer Graphics for Decision Making,"
1969   Harvard Business Review, vol. 47, November-
        December, pp. 121-132.

Miller, J.R., Professional Decision Making, N.Y.: Praeger
1971   Publishers.

Morris, W.T., The Analysis of Management Decisions, Home-
1964   wood, Ill.: Richard D. Irwin.

Morris, W.T., Management Science: A Bayesian Approach,
1968   Englewood Cliffs, N.J.: Prentice-Hall.

Morton, M., Management Decision Systems, Cambridge, Mass.:
1971   Harvard University Press.

Morton, M.S., and A.M. McCosh, "Terminal Costing for Better
1968   Decisions," Harvard Business Review, vol. 46,
        May-June, pp. 147-156.

Myers, B.L., and A.J. Melcher, "On the Choice of Risk
1969   Levels in Managerial Decision Making," Manage-
        ment Science, vol. 15, October, pp. 3-39.

Owen, J., "Criterion for Investing in Information,"
1968   Management Science, vol. 14, August, pp. 715-720.

Owens, B.D., "Decision Theory in Academic Administration,"
1968   Academy of Management Journal, vol. 11, June,
        pp. 221-232.

Pollock, S.M., "Minimum Cost Checking Using Imperfect In-
1967   formation," Management Science, vol. 13, March,
        pp. 454-465.

Pratt, J.W., et al., Introduction to Statistical Decision
1965   Theory, N.Y.: McGraw-Hill.

Prince, T., Information Systems for Management Planning
1966   and Control, Homewood, Ill.: Richard D. Irwin.

Quade, E.S., Analysis for Military Decisions, Chicago,
1964   Ill.: Rand McNally & Co.

Raiffa, H., Decision Analysis: Introductory Lectures on
1968   Choices Under Uncertainty, Reading, Mass.:
        Addison-Wesley.

Raiffa, H., and R. Schlaiffer, <u>Applied Statistical Decision</u>
1961   <u>Theory</u>, Cambridge, Mass.: Harvard Business
        School.

Reinke, W.A., "Mathematical Models for Decision-Making in
1971   Population and Family Planning," <u>American</u>
        <u>Journal of Public Health</u>, vol. 61, July, pp.
        1281-1284.

Reutlinger, S., <u>Techniques for Project Appraisal Under Un-</u>
1971   <u>certainty</u>, Baltimore: Johns Hopkins Press.

Richards, M. deV., <u>Management Decision Making</u>, Homewood,
1966   Ill.: Richard D. Irwin.

Richetto, G.M., "Organizations Circa 1990: Demise of the
1970   Pyramid," <u>Personnel Journal</u>, vol. 49, July,
        pp. 598-603.

Riter, J.C., "Merchandizing Decision Under Uncertainty,"
1967   <u>Journal of Marketing</u>, vol. 31, January, pp.
        44-47.

Roman, D.D., "Technological Forecasting in the Decision
1970   Process," <u>Academy of Management Journal</u>, vol.
        13, June, pp. 127-138.

Schlaiffer, R., <u>Analysis of Decisions Under Uncertainty</u>,
1967   N.Y.: McGraw-Hill.

Sciarrino, G., "Decision Theory and Scientific Method:
1967   Past, Present and Future," <u>Management Inter-</u>
        <u>national Review</u>, vol. 7, February, pp. 59-93.

Simon, H., <u>The Shape of Automation for Men and Management</u>,
1965   N.Y.: Harper & Row.

Simone, A.J., "A Dynamic Programming Approach to the Maxi-
1967   mization of Output from Production Processes of
        Varying Efficiencies," <u>Academy of Management</u>,
        June, pp. 129-143.

Skousen, K.F., and B.E. Needles, "Conceptual Framework
  1969   for Analyzing and Evaluating Managerial De-
          cisions," <u>National Association of Accountants
          Journal</u>, vol. 50, January, pp. 9-11.

Smith, C., "Consistency in Statistical Inference and De-
  1961   cision," <u>Royal Statistical Society Journal</u>,
          vol. 23, pp. 1-37.

Soelberg, P.O., "Unprogrammed Decision Making," <u>Industrial
  1967   Management Review</u>, vol. 18, Spring, pp. 19-29.

Spillane, E.J., "The Anatomy of a Decision," <u>Hospital
  1969   Progress</u>, vol. 50, April, pp. 47-50.

Spivey, W.A., "Decision Making and Probabilistic Program-
  1968   ming," <u>Industrial Management Review</u>, vol. 10,
          Winter, pp. 47-50.

Starr, M.K., "Discussion of some Normative Criteria for
  1966   Decision Making Under Uncertainty," <u>Industrial
          Management Review</u>, vol. 8, Fall, pp. 71-78.

Thiel, H., <u>Optimal Decision Rules for Government and
  1964   Industry</u>, Amsterdam: North Holland Publishing Co.

Walton, W.W., "Modern Decision Theory Applied to Medical
  1964   Diagnosis," Doctoral Dissertation, Johns
          Hopkins University, Dept. O.R. and I.E.

Weingart, S.R., "Understanding Management Decision Pro-
  1969   cesses," <u>Journal of Systems Management</u>, vol.
          20, April, pp. 37-39.

Weinwurm, E.H., "Preliminaries of the Decision Making
  1968   Process," <u>Management International Review</u>, vol.
          8, pp. 115-119.

Part 5.

DECISION MAKING, OBJECTIVES AND CONFLICT

Abernathy, W.J., and R.S. Rosenbloom, "Parallel Strategies
  1969   in Development Projects," Management Science,
          vol. 15, June, pp. 486-505.

Ackoff, R.L., Scientific Method: Optimizing Applied Research
  1962   Decisions, N.Y.: John Wiley & Sons.

Adelson, R.M., and J.M. Norman, "Operational Research and
  1969   Decision-Making," Operational Research Quarterly,
          vol. 20, December,pp. 399-420.

Alexis, M., and C.Z. Wilson, Organizational Decision Making,
  1967   Englewood Cliffs, N.J.: Prentice-Hall.

Bainbridge, L., et al., "Study of Real-Time Human Decision
  1968   Making Using a Plant Simulator," Operational
          Research Quarterly, vol. 19, April, pp. 91-106.

Basil, D., Executive Decision Making Through Simulation,
  1965   Columbus, Ohio: Charles E. Merrill, Publisher.

Becker, G., and C. McClintock, "Value Behavioral Decision
  1967   Theory," Annual Review of Psychology, vol. 18,
          pp. 239-286.

Bernan, J.C., "Choice Criteria, Decision Behavior, and
  1968   Personality," Journal of Marketing Research,
          vol. 5, May, pp. 155-164.

Blankenship, L.V., and R.E. Miles, "Organizational Structure
  1968   and Managerial Decision Behavior," Administra-
          tive Science Quarterly, vol. 13, June, pp. 106-
          120.

Brim, O., Jr., Personality and Decision Processes,
  1962   Stanford, Calif.: Stanford University Press.

Broadbent, D.E., "Aspects in Human Decision Making," Com-
  1968   puters and Automation, vol. 17, May, pp. 30-38.

Brown, R.E., Judgment in Administration, N.Y.: McGraw-
1965   Hill.

Bruns, W.J., "Accounting Information and Decision-Making:
1968   Some Behavioral Hypotheses," Accounting Review,
vol. 43, July, pp. 469-480.

Byrd, R.E., "How Much Risk Can you Afford to Take," Manage-
1971   ment Review, vol. 60, May, pp. 4-9.

Churchman, C.W., Prediction and Optimal Decision, Englewood
1961   Cliffs, N.J.: Prentice-Hall.

Churchman, C.W., Challenge to Reason, N.Y.: McGraw-Hill.
1968

Colby, R.M., "Computer Simulation of Change in Personal
1967   Belief Systems," Behavioral Science, vol. 12,
May, pp. 248-253.

Collier, A.T., Management Men and Values, N.Y.: Harper &
1962   Row.

Conrath, D.W., "Organizational Decision Making Behavior
1967   Under Varying Conditions of Uncertainty,"
Management Science, vol. 13, April, pp. 487-500.

Cooper, J., The Art of Decision Making, Garden City, N.Y.:
1961   Doubleday & Co.

Davis, M., and M.G. Weinbaum, Metropolitan Decision Pro-
1969   cesses, Chicago, Ill.: Rand McNally & Co.

Dickson, G.W., "Generalized Model of Administrative Deci-
1970   sions: An Experimental Test," Management Science,
vol. 17, September, pp. 35-47.

Dror, Y., Public Policymaking Reexamined, Chicago: Science
1968   Research Associates Distributors.

Drucker, P.F., Managing for Results, N.Y.: Harper & Row.
1964

Drucker, P.F., The Effective Executive, N.Y.: Harper & Row.
1967

Dutton, J.M., and R.E. Walton, "Interdepartmental Conflict
1966   and Cooperation: Two Contrasting Studies,"
        Human Organization, vol. 25, Fall, pp.207-220.

Edwards, W., "Behavioral Decision Theory," Annual Review
1961   of Psychology, vol. 12, pp. 473-498.

Edwards, W., Bibliography: Decision Making, Ann Arbor,
1964   Mich.: University of Michigan Press.

Fairhead, J., Exercises in Business Decisions, London:
1965   English University Press.

Ferber, R.C., "Role of the Subconscious in Executive Deci-
1967   sion Making," Management Science, vol. 13,
        April, pp. 519-532.

Ferber, R.C., "Dark Side of Decision-Making," Manage-
1971   ment Review, vol. 60, March, pp. 4-13.

Ference, T.P., "Organizational Communications Systems and
1970   the Decision Process," Management Science, vol.
        17, October, pp. 83-96.

Festinger, L., Conflict, Decision and Dissonance, Stanford,
1970   Calif.: Stanford University Press.

Fishburn, P.C., Decision and Value Theory, N.Y.: John
1964   Wiley & Sons.

Galanter, E., "The Direct Measurement of Utility and Sub-
1962   jective Probability," American Journal of
        Psychology, vol. 75, June, pp. 208-220.

Haire, M., et al., Managerial Thinking, N.Y.: John Wiley
1966   & Sons.

Hamilton, J., Decision Making in Hospital Administration
1960   and Medical Care, Minneapolis: University of
        Minnesota Press.

Hansell, N., et al., "Decision Counseling: Coping at
1971   Crisis-in-Transit," Current Psychiatric Thera-
        pies, vol. 11, pp. 129-138.

Hirsch, R.E., "Value of Information," <u>Journal of Account-</u>
1968   <u>ing</u>, vol. 125, June, pp. 41-45.

Hirsch, W.Z., "Input-Ouput Techniques for Urban Government
1968   Decisions," <u>American Economic Review</u>, vol. 48,
        May, pp. 162-170, 182-187.

Hough, L., <u>Modern Research for Administrative Decisions</u>,
1970   Englewood Cliffs, N.J.: Prentice-Hall.

Howard, J.A., and W.M. Morgenroth, "Information Processing
1968   Model of Executive Decisions," <u>Management</u>
        <u>Science</u>, vol. 14, March, pp. 416-428.

Hughes, C.L., <u>Goal Setting, Key to Individual and Organiza-</u>
1965   <u>tional Effectiveness</u>, N.Y.: American Management
        Association Press.

Johnson, R.J., <u>Executive Decisions</u>, Cincinnati, Ohio:
1963   South Western Publishing Co.

Kepner, C., and B.B. Tregde, <u>The Rational Manager</u>, N.Y.:
1965   McGraw-Hill.

Kernan, J.B., "Choice Criteria, Decision Behavior, and Per-
1968   sonality," <u>Journal of Marketing Research</u>, vol.
        5, May, pp. 155-164.

Marquis, D.G., "Individual and Group Decisions Involving
1968   Risk," <u>Industrial Management Review</u>, vol. 57,
        Spring, pp. 69-75.

Marschak, J., "Actual Versus Consistent Decision Behavior,"
1964   <u>Behavioral Science</u>, vol. 9, September, pp.103-110.

McCreary, E.A., "When a Decision is a Gamble: What is the
1967   Best Bet?" <u>Management Review</u>, vol. 56, June,
        pp. 37-44.

Miller, J.R., <u>Professional Decision Making</u>, N.Y.: Praeger
1971   Press.

Ofstad, H., <u>An Inquiry Into the Freedom of Decision</u>, N.Y.:
1961   Humanities.

Patterson, J.R., "Decision Making Applications of Direct
1968   Cost Information," <u>National Association of
        Accountants Journal</u>, vol. 49, January, pp.11-22.

Richards, M.deV., <u>Management Decision Making</u>, Homewood,
1966   Ill.: Richard D. Irwin.

Shrode, W.A., and W.B. Brown, "Study of Optimality in Re-
1970   current Decision-Making of Lower Level Managers,"
        <u>Academy of Management Journal</u>, vol. 13, December,
        pp. 389-401.

Shull, F., <u>Organizational Decision Making</u>, N.Y.: McGraw-
1970   Hill.

Siegel, S., et al., <u>Choice, Strategy and Utility</u>, N.Y.:
1964   McGraw-Hill.

Thometz, C., <u>The Decision Makers</u>, Dallas: Southern
1963   Methodist University Press.

Thompson, H.E., and W. Beranek, "Efficient Use of an Impor-
1966   tant Forecast," <u>Management Science</u>, vol. 13,
        November, pp. 233-243.

Thorneycroft, W.T., et al., "Investment Decisions Under
1968   Uncertainty and Variability--Some Practical Ex-
        periences of Using Forecasts and Probabilities,"
        <u>Operational Research Quarterly</u>, vol. 19, June,
        pp. 143-160.

Vickers, Sir G., <u>The Art of Judgement</u>, N.Y.: Basic Books.
1965

Weisselberg, R.C., and J.G. Cowley, "Strategies for Decision
1970   Making," <u>Management Services</u>, vol. 7, January,
        pp. 41-46.

Williams, J.D., "Study of a Decision Model for R. and D.
1969   Project Selection," <u>Operational Research Quarterly</u>
        vol. 20, September, pp. 361-373.

Ying, C.C., "Learning by Doing an Adaptive Approach to
1967   Multiperiod Decisions," Operations Research,
        vol. 15, September, pp. 797-812.

Ying, C.C., "Model of Adaptive Team Decision," Operations
1969   Research, vol. 17, September, pp. 800-811.

Young, J.P., "Information Nexus Guides Decision Systems,"
1966   Modern Hospital, vol. 106, February, pp. 101-105.

Part 6.

ASPECTS OF PLANNING

Abel-Smith, B., "Hospital Planning in Great Britain,"
1962   Hospitals, vol. 36, May 1, pp. 30-35.

Abel-Smith, B., An International Study of Health Expenditure
1967   and its Relevance for Health Planning, Geneva,
        Switzerland: World Health Organization.

Agnew, H.C., "Programming and Planning for Surgical Suites,"
1966   Proceedings of the American Association of Hos-
        pital Consultants, April 20.

American Association of Hospital Consultants, A.B. Mills
1969   (ed.), Functional Planning of General Hospitals,
        N.Y.: McGraw-Hill.

American Hospital Association, Manual of Hospital Planning
1966   Procedures, Chicago.

American Journal of Public Health, Committee on Environment
1968   of the American Public Health Association,
        "Environmental Factors in Health Planning," vol.
        58, February, pp. 358-359.

American Public Health Association, Self Study Guide for
1967   Community Health Action Planning, New York,
        July.

Ammer, D.S., "Side Effects of Planning," Harvard Business
1970   Review, vol. 48, May, pp. 32-34ff.

Anderson, N., and D. Anderson, Comprehensive Health Planning
1970   in the States--A Current Status Report, Minn.:
        American Rehabilitation Foundation.

Ardell, D.B., "Urban Planning and Health Planning Inter-
1969   relationships," American Journal of Public
        Health, vol. 59, no. 11, pp. 2051-2055.

Ardell, D.B., "CHP, Regional Councils and Public Interest:
1971   Case for New Leadership," Inquiry, vol. 8,
        December, pp. 27-35.

Arnold, M.F., "Basic Concepts and Crucial Issues in Health
1969   Planning," American Journal of Public Health,
        vol. 59, pp. 1686-1697.

Arnold, M.F., and D.L. Hink, "Agency Problems in Planning
1966   for Community Health Needs," Medical Care, vol.
        6, November-December, pp. 454-466.

Aronson, J.B., "Planning for Community Health Services,"
1964   Public Health Reports, vol. 79, no. 12, pp.
        1101-1106.

Astrachan, B.M., et al., "Systems Approach to Day Hospitali-
1970   zation," Archives of General Psychiatry, June,
        pp. 22, 550-559.

Badgley, R.F., "Studies in Planning Health Manpower: The
1971   Varma Meeting," Journal of Health and Social
        Behavior, vol. 12, March, pp. 4-10.

Baker, T.D., "Dynamics of Health Manpower Planning,"
1966   Journal of Medical Care, vol. 4, no. 4, pp.
        205-211.

Bartscht, K.G., "The Development of an Effective Method-
1965   ology for Determining Staffing Requirements in
        Hospitals," Project Report, Hospital Systems
        Research Group, Ann Arbor, Mich.: University
        of Michigan Press, February.

Beehler, P.J., "EDP: Simulating Systematic Corporate Plan-
1969   ning," Journal of Systems Management, vol. 20,
        November, pp. 26-31.

Bennett, A.C., "Requirements for Achieving Progress in
1970   Hospital Systems Engineering," Hospital Topics,
        vol. 48, February, pp. 50-54.

Berg, N., "Strategic Planning in Conglomerate Companies,"
1965   Harvard Business Review, May-June, pp. 79-92.

Berg, R.L., et al., "Bed Utilization Studies for Community
1969   Planning," Journal of the American Medical
        Association, vol. 207, no. 13, pp. 2411-2413.

Berg, R.L., et al., "Assessing the Health Care Needs of the
   1970   Aged," Health Services Research, vol. 5, Spring,
           pp. 36-59.

Berger, D.G., and E.A. Garder, "Uses of Community Surveys
   1971   in Mental Health Planning," American Journal of
           Physicians, vol. 61, January,p. 1104.

Berry, R.E., Jr., "Returns to Scale in the Production of
   1967   Hospital Services," Health Services Research,
           vol. 2, Summer, pp. 123-139.

Binstock, R.H., "The Politics of Health Planning, Effective
   1969   Planning Through Political Influence," American
           Journal of Public Health, vol. 59, no. 5, pp.
           808-813.

Blakely, R.T., 3rd., "Markov Models and Manpower Planning,"
   1970   Industrial Management Review, vol. 11, Winter,
           pp. 39-46.

Böer, G.B., "Extending the Hospital Planning Horizon,"
   1972   Hospital Administration, vol. 17, Winter,
           pp. 51-60.

Bolan, R.S., "Emerging Views of Planning," Journal of the
   1967   American Institute of Planners, vol. 33, July,
           pp. 233-245.

Bower, J.L., "Planning Within the Firm (with discussion),"
   1970   American Economic Review, vol. 60, May, pp.
           186-198.

Bowling, J.P., "Some Aspects of Mental Health Program
   1963   Planning Utilizing Management Systems Concepts,"
           Technical Paper 26, Operations Research, Inc.
           Silver Springs, Md., August.

Branch, M.C., Selected References for Corporate Planning,
   1966   N.Y.: American Management Association Press.

Breslow, L., "Political Jurisdictions, Voluntarism and
   1968   Health Planning," American Journal of Public
           Health, vol. 58, July, pp. 1147-1153.

Brotchie, J.F., "General Planning Model," Management
    1969   Science, vol. 16, November, pp. 265-269.

Brown, R.E., "Eight 'Whys' of Hospital Utilization,"
    1963   Canadian Hospital, June, pp. 58-61.

Bugbee, G., "How Many Hospital Beds Are Needed?" Hospital
    1963   Management, vol. 96, September, pp. 48-51.

Bulletin of the New York Academy of Medicine, "Planning for
    1968   Community Health Services: Perspectives for
            Action," vol. 44, February, pp. 83-219.

Callan, L.B., "Health Education Aid Trainee Project,"
    1969   Public Health Reports, vol. 84, May, pp. 459-464.

Cantley, M.F., "Long-Range Planning Case Study," Operations
    1969   Research Quarterly, vol. 20, April, pp. 7-20.

Carithers, R.W., "Area Wide Planning Accomplishments and
    1964   Abstacles," Hospital Progress, December, pp.
            81-84, 106.

Chambers, J.C., et al., "Catalytic Agent for Effective
    1971   Planning," Harvard Business Review, January-
            February, pp. 110-119.

Chicago University Center for Health Administration,
    1969   Selected Papers on Health Planning: Its Purposes,
            Evaluating Outcomes, Chicago.

Coe, R.M., Planned Change in the Hospital, N.Y.: Praeger
    1970   Publishers.

Colt, A.M., "Elements of Comprehensive Health Planning,"
    1970   American Journal of Public Health, vol. 60, no.
            7, pp. 1194-1204.

Connors, E.J., "Measuring Hospital Effectiveness--Manage-
    1969   ment Patterns," University of Michigan Medical
            Center Journal, vol. 35, April-June, pp. 35,
            116-118.

Cooke, J.E., "Needs of Employee in the Computerized Hos-
    1968   pital," Canadian Hospital, March, pp. 50-53.

Council on Medical Service, "Comprehensive Planning of
    1968   Health Facilities and Services," Journal of
            the American Medical Association, vol. 204,
            no. 9, pp. 808-810.

Daniels, R., et al., "An Example of Sub-regional Health
    1970   Planning," Inquiry, vol. 7, December, pp. 25-33.

Densen, P.M., et al., "Research, Program Planning and Evalu-
    1966   ation," Public Health Reports, vol. 81, January,
            pp. 49-96.

Dickey, W.J., et al., "Comprehensive Health Planning--
    1970   Federal, State, Local: Concepts and Realities,"
            Wisconsin Law Review, 1970, pp. 839-878.

Durbin, R.L.,and W.H.Springhall, Organization and Adminis-
    1969   tration of Health Care: Theory, Practice,
            Environment, St. Louis, Mo.: C.V. Mosby Co.

DuVall, W.L., "Consumer Participation in Health Planning,"
    1971   Hospital Administration, vol. 16, Fall, pp.
            35-49.

Elling, R.H., "Health Planning in International Perspec-
    1971   tive," Medical Care, vol. 9, May-June, pp.
            214-234.

Engel, A., et al., "Areawide Planning of Health Services,"
    1968   World Hospitals, vol. 4, October, pp. 212-225.

Ewing, D.W., The Practice of Planning, N.Y.: Harper & Row.
    1968

Ewing, D.W., The Human Side of Planning: Tool or Tyrant?
    1969   N.Y.: Macmillan.

Feingold, E., "The Politics of Health Planning: The Chang-
    1969   ing Political Character of Health Planning,"
            American Journal of Public Health, vol. 59, no.
            5, pp. 803-808.

Fifer, E.Z., "Hang-ups in Health Planning," American Jour-
    1969   nal of Public Health, vol. 59, May, pp. 765-769.

Flagle, C.D., "Communication and Control in Comprehensive
1969   Patient Care and Health Planning," Annals of
The New York Academy of Sciences, vol. 161,
September 30, pp. 714-729.

Frazier, T.M., "The Questionable Role of Statistics in Com-
1970   prehensive Health Planning," American Journal
of Physicians, vol. 60, no. 9, pp. 1701-1705.

Freiburn, R.B., "Two Years Invested in Planning New Loyola
1969   Information System," Modern Hospital, vol.
112, February, pp. 99-100.

Friedman, J., "A Conceptual Model for the Analysis of
1967   Planning Behavior," Administrative Science
Quarterly, vol. 12, September, pp. 225-257.

Getting, V.A., "Planning, Implementation and Evaluation of
1964   Community Health Services," Canadian Journal
of Public Health, vol. 55, p. 517.

Gottlieb, S.R., "How Hospital Planners and City Planners
1967   Work Together," Hospitals, vol. 41, September
1, pp. 65-68.

Haggerty, J.R., "Planning Computerized Information System,"
1970   Hospitals, vol. 44, pp. 43-46.

Hallquist, B., "A Frontrunner in Facility Planning,"
1970   Industrial Developments, vol. 139, January,
pp. 12-13.

Hardy, O.B., "Systematic Processes Applied to Health Care
1971   Planning," Hospital Administration, vol. 16,
Winter, pp. 7-24.

Hilleboe, H.E., "Health Planning on a Community Basis,"
1968   Medical Care, vol. 6, May-June, pp. 203-214.

Hilleboe, H.E., and M. Schaefer, "Administrative Require-
1968   ments for Comprehensive Health Planning at the
State Level," American Journal of Public
Health, vol. 58, June, pp. 1039-1046.

Hilleboe, H.E., and M. Schaefer, "Papers and Bibliography
    1967   on Community Health Planning," Graduate
            School of Public Affairs, Albany, N.Y.: State
            University of New York, August.

Hilton, P., <u>Planning Corporate Growth and Diversification</u>,
    1970   N.Y.: McGraw-Hill.

Hochbaum, G.M., "Consumer Participation in Health Planning:
    1969   Toward Conceptual Clarification," <u>American</u>
            <u>Journal of Public Health</u>, vol. 59, no. 9, pp.
            1698-1705.

Holder, L., and O.L. Deniston, "A Decision Making Approach
    1968   to Comprehensive Health Planning," <u>Public</u>
            <u>Health Reports</u>, vol. 83, no. 7, pp. 559-568.

Horvath, W.J., "Need for Estimating the Influence of Tech-
    1968   nological and Social Changes on Future Health
            Facility Requirements," <u>Health Services Re-</u>
            <u>search</u>, vol. 3, Spring, pp. 3-9.

Hudenbury, R., <u>Planning the Community Hospital</u>, N.Y.:
    1967   McGraw-Hill.

Hunter, R., and J. Schnee, "Long Range Planning in Mental
    1966   Health," <u>Management Science</u>, vol. 12, June,
            pp. B 519-B 522.

Jacobs, A.R., and R.B. Froh, "Significance of Public Law
    1968   89-749 Comprehensive Health Planning," <u>New</u>
            <u>England Journal of Medicine</u>, vol. 279, Decem-
            ber, pp. 1314-1318.

Jacobs, W.F., Jr., "Comprehensive Health Planning Problems
    1969   and Benefits," <u>Hospital Progress</u>, November,
            pp. 67-68, 69, 88.

Jamison, R.E., "Councils of Governments as the Areawide
    1971   Comprehensive Health Planning Agency," <u>Ameri-</u>
            <u>can Journal of Public Health</u>, vol. 61, November,
            pp. 2240-2245.

Johnson, E.T., "The Delivery of Health Care in the Ghetto,"
1969   National Medical Association, vol. 6, May,
        pp. 263-270.

Jongerius, T.I., "A Middle-Management Development Program
1969   for Hospitals," Canadian Hospital, January,
        pp. 40-43.

Kane, D.A., "Comprehensive Health Planning: A Study in
1969   Creative Federalism," American Journal of
        Public Health, vol. 59, no. 9, pp. 1706-1712.

Kissick, W.L., "Forecasting Health Manpower Needs: The
1967   Numbers Game is Obsolete," Hospitals, vol. 41,
        September 16, pp. 47-51.

Kissick, W.L., "Effective Utilization: The Critical Factor
1968   in Health Manpower," American Journal of Public
        Health, vol. 58, January, pp. 23-29.

Klarman, H.E., "Some Technical Problems in Areawide Planning
1964   for Hospital Care," Journal of Chronic Disease,
        vol. 17, no. 9, pp. 735-757.

Levin, R.J., and C.A. Kirkpatrick, Planning and Control with
1966   PERT/CPM, N.Y.: McGraw-Hill.

Llewelyn-Davies, R., and H.M.C. Macaulay, Hospital Planning
1966   and Administration, Geneva, Switzerland: World
        Health Organization.

Long, M., "Efficient Use of Hospitals," in The Economics
1964   of Health and Medical Care, Ann Arbor: Univer-
        sity of Michigan Press. pp. 211-226.

Lubin, J.W., et al., "Highway Network Minimum Path Selection
1965   Applied to Health Facility Planning," Public
        Health Reports, vol. 80, no. 9, pp. 771-778.

Mattison, B.F., "Community Health Planning and the Profes-
1968   sions Health," American Journal of Public
        Health, vol. 58, no. 6, pp. 1015-1021.

May, J.J., <u>Health Planning: Its Past Potential</u>, Chicago,
     1967   Ill.: University of Chicago, Center for Health
             Administration Studies.

McFarlan, F.W., "Problems in Planning the Information
     1971   System," <u>Harvard Business Review</u>, vol. 49,
             March-April, pp. 75-89.

Michael, J.M., et al., "Basic Information Systems for Health
     1968   Planning," <u>Public Health Reports</u>, vol. 83, no.
             1, pp. 21-28.

Miller, E., <u>Advanced Techniques for Strategic Planning</u>,
     1970   N.Y.: American Management Association Press.

Mills, A.B., <u>Functional Planning of a General Hospital</u>,
     1964   N.Y.: McGraw-Hill.

Mockler, R.J., "Theory and Practice of Planning," <u>Harvard</u>
     1970   <u>Business Review</u>, vol. 48, March, pp. 148+.

Morris, R., "The City of the Future and Planning for Health,"
     1968   <u>American Journal of Public Health</u>, vol. 52,
             January, pp. 13-22.

Muller, C., "Health at What Price? Some Notes for Compre-
     1969   hensive Health Planners," <u>American Journal of</u>
             <u>Public Health</u>, vol. 59, April, pp. 651-656.

Navarro, V., "Planning Personal Health Services, A Markovian
     1969   Model," <u>Medical Care</u>, vol. 7, no. 3, pp. 242-
             249.

Navarro, V., "The City and the Region," <u>American Behavioral</u>
     1971   <u>Science</u>, vol. 14, July-August, pp. 865-892.

Newton, R.G., and D.J. Spurrell, "A Development of Multiple
     1967   Regression for the Analysis of Routine Data,"
             <u>Applied Statistics</u>, vol. 16, pp. 51-64.

Peloquin, E.J., "Catalytic Comprehensive Health Planning,"
     1971   <u>American Journal of Public Health</u>, vol. 61,
             October, pp. 1979-1982.

Perloff, H.S. (ed., with assistance of E. Foster and P.
1961   Norton), Planning and the Urban Community,
        Pittsburgh, Pa.: Carnegie Institute of Tech-
        nology.

Pill, J., "Delphi Method: Substance, Context, a Critique
1971   and an Annotated Bibliography," Socio-Economic
        Planning Sciences, vol. 5, February, pp. 57-71.

Rosenthal, G.C., Hospital Utilization in the United States,
1964   Chicago: American Hospital Association. pp.
        55-62.

Runck, H.M., "Computer Planning for Hospitals: The Large-
1969   Scale Education and Involvement of Employees,"
        Computers and Automation, June 1, pp. 33-35.

Ryder, C.F., et al., "Patient Assessment, An Essential Tool
1971   in Placement and Planning Care," HSMHA Health
        Reports, vol. 86, October, pp. 923-932.

Sarnoff, R.W., "In Praise of Planning a Proposal for Testing
1970   the Systems Approach to Social Problems," Con-
        ference Board Record, vol. 7, February, pp. 45-47.

Saxberg, B.O., and J.W. Slocum, Jr., "The Management of
1968   Scientific Manpower," Management Science, vol.
        14, pp. B 473-B 489.

Schneider, J.B., "A New Approach to Areawide Planning of
1968   Metropolitan Hospital Systems," Hospitals,
        vol. 42, April 16, pp. 79-83.

Schrager, L., Planning for Better Health Services: Guide-
1970   lines and Criteria for Planning Hospital and
            Related Health Services in New York City, Health
            and Hospital Planning Council of Southern New
            York, May.

Sibley, H., "How a Planning Council Evaluates Hospital De-
1964   velopment Proposals," Hospital Management,
        vol. 98, October, pp. 53-55, 116.

Sigmond, R.M., "Process of Outcome Planning--Which Concept
1969   Will Dominate?" Hospital Topics, June, pp. 12-14.

Somers, H.M., and A.R. Somers, <u>Doctors, Patients and Health</u>
1961   <u>Insurance</u>, Washington, D.C.: Brookings Institute.

Sparks, J.E., "Planning Health Services," <u>Canadian Journal</u>
1964   <u>of Public Health</u>, vol. 55, p. 117.

Spiegel, H., "Health Planning in the Context of Comprehen-
1968   sive Community Development," <u>Bulletin New York</u>
<u>Academy of Medicine</u>, vol. 44, February, pp.
199-203.
Starr, M.K., "Planning Models," <u>Management Science</u>, vol.
1966   13, December, pp. 115-141.

Stevens, C.M., and G.D. Brown, "Market Structure Approach to
1971   Health-Manpower 'Planning'," <u>American Journal</u>
<u>of Public Health</u>, vol. 61, October, pp. 1988-
1995.

Storck, J., "Hard Facts for Health Planning," <u>Public Health</u>
1968   <u>Reports</u>, vol. 83, October, pp. 841-848.

Strauss, M., "Health Care Planning," <u>Hospitals</u>, vol. 43,
1969   April 1, pp. 105-108.

Strauss, M., and I. deGroot, "Bookshelf on Community Planning
1971   for Health," <u>American Journal of Public Health</u>,
vol. 61, April, pp. 656-679.

Tilles, S., "Strategies for Allocating Funds," <u>Harvard</u>
1966   <u>Business Review</u>, January-February, pp. 72-80.

Thoren, B.J., et al., "Attitude Study, Training Help Employ-
1969   ees Adapt to Use of Computers," <u>Hospitals</u>,
March 1, vol. 43, pp. 61-64.

Thurston, P.H., "Make Technological Forecasting Serve Cor-
1971   porate Planning," <u>Harvard Business Review</u>,
vol. 49, September-October, pp. 98-102.

U.S. Public Health Service, with State and Territorial
1967   Health Planning Agencies, "Partnership for
Health," <u>Special Conferences of the Surgeon</u>
<u>General</u>, Washington, D.C., June 12.

Vancil, R.F., "Accuracy of Long-Range Planning," <u>Harvard</u>
1970   <u>Business Review</u>, vol. 48, September, pp. 98-101.

Vietorisz, T., "Quantized Preferences and Planning by Prio-
1970   rities," <u>American Economic Review</u>, vol. 60,
        March, pp. 65-69.

Wagle, G., "Use of Models for Environmental Forecasting and
1969   Corporate Planning," <u>Operations Research</u>, vol.
        20, September, pp. 327-336.

Weber, M.M., "Comprehensive Planning and Social Responsibi-
1963   lity," <u>American Institute of Planning</u>, vol. 29,
        November, pp. 232-241.

Weil, T.P., et al., "Coordinating Health and Management
1967   Knowledge for the Training of Health Managers,"
        <u>Journal of Medical Education</u>, vol. 42, August,
        pp. 759-764.

Wenkert, W., et al., "Concepts and Methodology: Planning
1968   Patient Care Services," <u>Medical Care</u>, vol. 7,
        July-August, pp. 327-331.

White, K.L., and J.H. Murnaghan, "Health Services Planning:
1970   Models and Means," <u>Health Services Research</u>,
        vol. 5, Winter, pp. 304-307.

Wirick, G.C., "A Multiple Equation Model of Demand for
1966   Health Care," <u>Health Services Research</u>, vol. 1,
        Winter, pp. 301-346.

Wirick, G.C., and R. Barlow, "The Economic and Social De-
1964   terminants of the Demand for Health Services,"
        in <u>Economics of Health and Medical Care</u>, Ann
        Arbor, Michigan: University of Michigan Press,
        pp. 95-124.

Wisowaty, K.W., et al., "Health Facilities Planning," <u>Jour-</u>
1964   <u>nal of the American Medical Association</u>, vol.
        190, pp. 752-756.

<u>World Health Organization</u>, "National Health Planning in
1967   Developing Countries," Series 350.

Yoder, F.D., and S. Reed, "Health Planning in Illinois, A
    1970   Case in Point," Archives of Environmental
            Health, vol. 20, no. 1, pp. 131-136.

Part 7.

PLANNING, PROGRAMMING AND BUDGETING

Ammer, D.S., "Recognizing Economic Indicators," Hospital
1969   Progress, October, pp. 25-29.

Anderson, O.W., and D. Neuhauser, "Rising Costs are Inher-
1969   ent in Modern Health Care Systems," Hospitals,
vol. 43, February, pp. 50-52.

Bahn, R., "Federal Budget Process," Public Health Reports,
1969   vol. 84, February, pp. 149-155.

Balls, H.R., "Planning, Programming, Budgeting in Canada,"
1970   in "New Techniques in Government Budgeting,"
Public Administration, vol. 48, October, pp.
289-305.

Bauer, R.W., "Try a New Approach to Planning," Hospital
1971   Financial Management, vol. 25, June, pp. 3-9.

Berkowitz, M.,"Planning, Programming, Budgeting and Systems
1968   Analysis: State-wide Planning and the Goals of
Vocational Rehabilitation," American Journal of
Public Health, vol. 58, September, pp. 1633-
1637.

Berry, R.E., J., "Returns to Scale in the Production of
1967   Hospital Services," Health Services Research,
Summer, pp. 123-139.

Boddy, F.A., "Cost-effectiveness, Cost-benefit Analysis
1971   and the Use of Audiovisual Resources," Scottish
Medical Journal, vol. 16, January, pp. 117-119.

Botner, S.B., "Four Years of PPBS: An Appraisal," Public
1970   Administration Review, vol. 30, July-August,
pp. 423-431.

Capron, W.M., "PPB and State Budgeting," Public Administra-
1969   tion Review, vol. 29, March-April, pp. 155-167.

Dean, A.L., "Planning, Programming and Budgeting in the U.S."
    1969   Management in Government, vol. 1, October-
            December, pp. 67-80.

Densen, P.M., G. James, and E. Cohart, "Research, Program
    1966   Planning and Evaluation," Public Health Re-
            ports, vol. 81, January, pp. 49-56.

Dyer, J.S., "Use of PPBS in a Public System of Higher Edu-
    1970   cation: Is it Cost-Effective?" Academy of
            Management Journal, vol. 13, September, pp. 285-
            299.

Feldstein, P.J., "An Empirical Investigation of the Marginal
    1961   Cost of Hospital Services," Graduate Program in
            Hospital Administration, Chicago, Ill.: Univer-
            sity of Chicago.

Fields, D.S., "Cost Effectiveness Analysis: Its Tasks and
    1966   Their Interrelation," Operations Research,
            May-June, vol. 14, pp. 515-527.

Fisher, G.H., "The World of Program Budgeting," The RAND
    1966   Corp., P. 3361, May.

Fitzpatrick, T.B., S.R. Gottlieb, and G.C. Wirick, "The
    1964   Nature of Hospital Costs," Ann Arbor: Bureau
            of Hospital Administration, University of
            Michigan.

Fletcher, T.W., "A New Look at Budgeting," Public Manage-
    1964   ment, vol. 46, February, pp. 26-28.

Fox, P.D., "A Theory of Cost Effectiveness for Military
    1965   System Analysis," Operations Research, vol. 13,
            March-April, pp. 191-201.

Gerwin, D., "Towards a Theory of Public Budgetary Decision-
    1969   Making," Administrative Science Quarterly,
            vol. 14, March, pp. 33-46.

Gorham, W.,   "Sharpening the Knife that Cuts the Public Pie:
    1968   Health, Education, and Welfare's Planning-
            Programming-Budgeting System," Public Adminis-
            stration Review, vol. 28, May-June, pp. 236-241.

Greenhouse, S.M., "The PPB System: Rationale, Language and
    1966   Idea Relationships," Public Administration
            Review, vol. 26, December, pp. 271-277.

Greenhouse, S.M., "Distributed Output Concept for the Plan-
    1967   ning-Programming-Budgeting System," Personnel
            Administration, vol. 30, July, pp. 35-51.

Gross, E., "When Occupations Meet: Professions in Trouble,"
    1967   Hospital Administration, vol. 12, no. 3, pp.
            40-59.

Lyden, F.J., and E.G. Miller, Planning, Programming, Bud-
    1968   geting: Selected Readings, Chicago, Ill.:
            Markham Publishing Co.

MacLeod, R.K., "Program Budgeting Works in Nonprofit Insti-
    1971   tutions: Mental Health Center in Massachusetts,"
            Harvard Business Review, vol. 49, September-
            October, pp. 46-56.

Marshall, A.W., "Cost-Benefit Analysis in Health," The
    1965   RAND Corp. P. 3274, December.

Michaeleen, Sister M., "Financial Planning," Hospital Pro-
    1964   gress, April, pp. 90-93.

Moore, T., "CCHPA Pushes for Change in Health System and
    1970   Costs," Hospital Progress, March, pp. 24-26.

Muller, C., "Health at What Price? Some Notes for Compre-
    1969   hensive Health Planners," American Journal of
            Public Health, vol. 59, April, pp. 651-656.

Mushkin, S.J., The Economics of Health and Medical Care,
    1964   Ann Arbor, Michigan: Bureau of Public Health
            Economics, University of Michigan.

Mushkin, S.J., "PPB in Cities," <u>Public Administration Re-</u>
     1969   <u>view</u>, vol. 29, March-April, pp. 167-178.

Page, D.A., "The Federal Planning-Programming-Budgeting
     1967   System," <u>American Institute of Planners Journal</u>,
             vol. 33, July, pp. 256-259.

Pan, L., "Planned Program Budgeting: A Workshop Report,"
     1971   <u>Nursing Outlook</u>, vol. 19, October, pp. 656-658.

Peters, G.H., "Cost Benefit Analysis and Public Expendi-
     1966   tures," <u>Eaton Paper 8</u>, The Institute of Econ-
             omic Affairs, London.

"Planning-Programming-Budgeting System: A Symposium,"
     1966   <u>Public Administration Review</u>, vol. 26, Decem-
             ber, pp. 243-310.

"Planning-Programming-Budgeting System Re-examined: Devel-
     1969   opment, Analysis, and Criticism, A Symposium,"
             <u>Public Administration Review</u>, vol. 29, March-
             April, pp. 111-202.

Posner, B., "Planning-Programming-Budgeting: A Financial
     1966   Management Approach," <u>Federal Accountant</u>, vol.
             15, Summer, pp. 9-21.

Priest, A.R., and R. Turvey, "Cost Benefit Analysis, A Sur-
     1965   vey," <u>Economic Journal</u>, December, pp. 683-735.

Proxmire, W., "PPBS--A New Approach to Government Spending,"
     1969   <u>Banking</u>, vol. 61, February, pp. 39-92.

Rice, D.P., "Estimating the Cost of Illness," <u>Health</u>
     1966   <u>Economic Series, No.5</u>, U.S. Public Health
             Service, May.

Savas, E.S., and L.L. Burkholz, <u>Cost and Effectiveness of</u>
     1968   <u>a System of Dispersed Ambulances</u>, New York:
             Office of Administration, Office of the Mayor.

Seccombe, E.W.C., "Analysis of Health Service Projects
     1970   Using Cost-Benefit Analysis," <u>World Hospitals</u>,
             vol. 6, October, pp. 214-221.

Smith, R.H., "Solution to Medical Accounting Problems,"
   1967   <u>Management Services</u>, July-August, pp. 28-33.

Spindler, A., "Planning, Programming and Budgeting System
   1969   and Social and Rehabilitation Services," <u>Wel-
            fare Review</u>, vol. 7, March-April, pp. 22-28.

Wachs, M.W., "Planning-Programming-Budgeting and Manage-
   1969   ment Information Systems for Mental Health,"
            <u>American Journal of Public Health</u>, vol. 59,
            February, pp. 261-266.

Weisbrod, B.A., "Some Problems in Pricing and Resource
   1965   Allocation in a Non-profit Industry--The Hospi-
            tals," <u>Journal of Business</u>, vol. 38, January,
            pp. 18-28.

Wildavsky, A., "The Political Economy of Efficiency: Cost
   1966   Benefit Analysis, Systems Analysis and Program
            Budgeting," <u>Public Administration Review</u>, vol.
            26, December, pp. 292-310.

Wiseman, J., "Cost Benefit Analysis and Health Service
   1963   Policy," <u>Scottish Journal Political Economy,</u>
            vol. 10, February, pp. 128-149.

Zimmer, W., et al., "Budget Planning: How Planning, Program-
   1971   ming, and Budgeting Systems Can be Useful to
            Associations," <u>Association Management</u>, vol. 23,
            November, pp. 40-43.

Part 8.

HEALTH INFORMATION SYSTEMS

Abrams, M.E., Medical Computing, N.Y.: American Elsevier
1970   Publishing Co.

Ackoff, R.L., "Management Misinformation Systems," Manage-
1967   ment Science, vol. 14, December, pp. B 147-B 156.

Allen, S.I., et al., "Use of Time Shared General-Purpose
1966   File Handling System in Hospital Research,"
        Proceedings of the IEEE, vol. 54, pp. 1641-1648.

Allen, S.I., and M. Otten, "The Telephone as a Computer In-
1969   put-Output Terminal for Medical Information,"
        Journal of the American Medical Association, vol.
        208, April 28, pp. 673-679.

Altman, M., "The Hospital Electronic Metamorphosis," Hospi-
1969   tals, vol. 43, December 1, pp. 42-45.

Amsterdam, D., and S. Schneierson, "Electronic Data Proces-
1969   sing for the Clinical Microbiology Laboratory,"
        Applied Microbiology, vol. 17, January, pp. 93-97.

Anand, H., "Computer-Based Hospital Information System:
1971   Ottawa Civic Hospital," Hospital Administration
        in Canada, vol. 13, September, pp. 46+.

Andrews, J., "Inventory Control in the Dietary Department,"
1969   Hospitals, vol. 43, October 1, pp. 96-99.

Andrews, J., "Estimating Food Costs by Computer," Hospi-
1969   tals, vol. 43, October, pp. 107-108.

Andrews, J., and H. B. Tuthill, "Computer-Based Management
1968   of Dietary Departments," Hospitals, vol. 42,
        July 16, pp. 117-123.

Anthony, J.M., Jr., "Data Processing in a Community of
1969   Hospitals," Hospital Progress, vol. 50, June,
        p. 64.

Anthony, R.N., Business Systems, Systems and Procedures
1966   Association.

Anthony, R.N., Design of Real-Time Computers Systems, N.Y.:
1967   Prentice-Hall.

Ausman, K.R., and V.E. Nicklas, "Administrators Study Com-
1967.   puter Applications in Hospital Setting," Hospi-
         tals, vol. 41, April. 16, pp. 44-45.

Automated Multiphasic Health Testing: Bibliography. U.S.
1970   Department of Health, Education and Welfare,
         Public Health Service, Washington, D.C., Govern-
         ment Printing Office, May.

Averill, B.W., "Use of Automated Information Systems in the
1970   Management and Evaluation of College Health Pro-
         grams," Journal of the American College Health
         Association, vol. 19, October, pp. 67-74.

Baird, H.W., and J.M. Garfunkel, "Electronic Data Process-
1965   ing of Medical Records," New England Journal of
         Medicine, vol. 272, June 10, pp. 1211-1215.

Ball, M.J., "Overview of Total Medical Information Systems,"
1971   Methods of Information in Medicine, vol. 10,
         April, pp.73-82.

Barker, K.N., "A Practical Philosophy for Hospital Data
1969   Processing," Hospitals, vol. 43, May 16, pp.
         69-71.
Barker, K.N., and W.E. McConnell, "The Problem of Detecting
1962   Medication Errors in Hospitals," American Journal
         of Hospital Pharmacy, vol. 19, August, pp. 360-369.

Barnett, G.O., Report to the Computer Research Study Section,
1966   National Institutes of Health, Laboratory of Com-
         puter Science, Massachusetts General Hospital
         (mimeographed), p. 16.

Barnett, G.O., An Annotated Selected Bibliography on the
1967   Application of Computers to Patient Care, Report
         from Laboratory of Computer Science, Boston,
         Mass.: Massachusetts General Hospital.

Barnett, O.G., and J.J. Baruch, <u>Hospital Computer Project,</u>
   1966   <u>Status Report</u>, Memo No. 9, Boston, Mass.:
            Massachusetts General Hospital.

Barnett, O.G., and P.A. Castleman, "Time Sharing Computer
   1967   System for Patient Care Activities," <u>Computer</u>
            <u>and Biomedical Research</u>, vol. 1, March, pp. 41-51.

Barnett, O.G., and R.A. Greenes, "Hospital Information Sys-
   1972   tems: Interface Problem, Conf. Proc. on use of
            Data Mechanization and Computers in Medicine,"
            <u>Annals New York Academy of Science</u>. (in press.)

Bartel, G.J., and J.J. Fahley, "Nursing Station is Home
   1969   Base for Phone-Printer System," <u>Modern Hospital</u>,
            vol. 113, November, pp. 85-88.

Bartsch, V., "Linking Analyzer with Computer Speeds Report-
   1967   ing of Lab Results," <u>Hospital Topics</u>, vol. 45,
            October, pp. 71-74.

Baruch, J.J., and O.G. Barnett, "Joint Ventures at Massa-
   1965   chusetts General," <u>Datamation</u>, vol. 11, Decem-
            ber, pp. 29-33.

Bellamy, C.J., and D. Race, "Computers and Medicine,"
   1968   <u>Australian Computer Journal</u>, May, pp. 78-81.

Bellchalmers, L.A., et al., "Computer-Assisted Method for
   1969   Compiling a Blood Group Register," <u>The Journal</u>
            <u>of Clinical Pathology</u>, vol. 22, March, pp. 229-
            232.

Bement, K.T., "Toward Complete Management Information Sys-
   1963   tems," <u>Systems and Procedures Journal</u>, vol. 14-15,
            September-October, pp. 36-39.

Bennett, W.L., and J. Houck, "A Three Step Plan for Automa-
   1967   mation," <u>Hospitals</u>, vol. 41, May 1, pp. 61-66.

Bennett, W.L., et al., "A Patient-Centered Hospital Infor-
   1969   mation System," <u>The Office</u>, vol. 69, May, pp.
            65-68.

Benson, D.R., "Computer Guide for Hospitals," Hospital
1968   Progress, vol. 49, November, pp. 63-65, 84.

Bergman, J.H., and D.L. Steffey, "Data Processing Improves
1969   Outpatient Management," Hospitals, vol. 43,
          January 1, pp. 49-51.

Berkley, C., "Case Histories--Untapped Medical Information
1965   Resource," American J.M. Electronics, (Supp.)
          vol. 4, July, pp. 4-5.

Berlin, M.M., "Computers in the Laboratory," Computers
1970   and Automation, vol. 19, June, pp. 24-27.

Blain, G., "The Computer is Here: Systems Development is
1969   Needed Now," Canadian Hospital, vol. 46, Septem-
          ber, pp. 40-42.

Blanco, J., Jr., "Streamlined Billing for Medicare Out-
1969   patients," Hospitals, vol. 43, August 1, pp.
          50-52.

Blankenship, T., "Computerized Accounting, Laboratory and
1969   Radiation Therapy Departments," Hospital Progress,
          vol. 50, July, pp. 62-64.

Blumberg, M.S., "Hospital Automation: The Needs and the
1961   Prospects," Hospitals, vol. 35, August 1, pp.
          34-43.

Blumenthal, S.C., Management Information Systems, Englewood,
1969   Cliffs, N.J.: Prentice-Hall.

Bogod, J.L., "Computer Applications in Hospitals," Indus-
1967   trial Electronics, March, pp. 98-103.

Bonney, J.B., Jr., "Perceptive Feedback," Data Processing
1964   Magazine, vol. 6, August, pp. 11-15.

Bower, J.B., and W. Welke (eds.), Financial Information
1968   Systems, Boston, Mass.: Houghton, Mifflin Co.

Bowman, J.L., and E.M. Brennan, "Computer-Assisted Menu
1969   Planning Provides Control of Food," Hospitals,
        vol. 42, August 16, p. 10.

Bove, J.R., and K.D. McKay, "Computer Approach to Hospital
1969   Blood Bank Inventory Control," Transfusion, vol.
        9, May-June, pp. 143-150.

Boyd, D.F., and H.S. Krasnow, "Economic Evaluation of
1963   Management Information Systems," IBM Journal,
        vol. 2, March.

Boyle, J.A., et al., "Construction of Model for Computer
1966   Assisted Diagnosis: Application to Problem of
        Non-Toxic Goiter," Quarterly Journal of Medi-
        cine, vol. 35, October, pp. 565-588.

Brisbane, H.M., "Building a Computer Assisted Nutrient
1969   File," Hospitals, vol. 43, November 22, pp. 92-
        96.

Brittin, G.M., and M. Werner, Automation and Data Processing
1970   in the Clinical Laboratory, Springfield, Ill.:
        Charles C. Thomas.

Brown, R.M., "Estimating Dietary Labor by Use of Work
1969   Modules," Hospitals, vol. 43, October 16, pp.
        103-106.

Bruce, R.A., and S.R. Yarnall, "Computer Aided Diagnosis
1966   of Cardiovascular Disorders," Journal of Chronic
        Diseases, vol. 19, pp. 473-484.

Bryan, D.J., et al., "Profile of Admission Chemical Data
1966   by Multi-Channel Automation: Evaluative Experi-
        ment," Clin. Chem., vol. 12, pp. 137-143.

Budd, P.J., "ADP as Aid in Personnel Shortage: Enables
1969   Better Use of Professionals," Hospital Topics,
        vol. 47, April, pp. 47-52.

Buchan, J.R., "New Approaches Needed," Hospitals, vol.
1970   44, May 16, pp. 99-102.

Caceres, C.A., and D.R. Barnes, "Computerized Care," Hospi-
1969   tals, vol. 43, December 1, pp. 49-52.

Caceres, C.A., and A.E. Rikli, Diagnostic Computers, Spring-
1969   field, Ill.: Charles C. Thomas.

Cammarn, M.R., "Computerized Records Provide Audit of Clinic
1968   Patient Care," Hospitals, vol. 42, September 1,
        pp. 74-79.

Cammarn, M.R., "Computer Systems Spread to Patient Care,"
1969   Modern Hospital, vol. 113, November, pp. 84-85.

Casbergue, J.P., "Health Professionals Need Education for
1969   Their Role in Automation," Hospital Topics, vol.
        47, May, pp. 42-44.

Chuang, Y.A., et al., "An Automation Analysis Approach to
1967   the Study of Neural Nets," Computers Biomedical
        Research, vol. 1, pp. 173-186.

Churchill, N.C., "Computer-Based Information Systems for
1969   Management: A Survey," National Association of
        Accountants.

Collen, M.F., "General Requirements for a Medical Infor-
1970   mation System," Computers and Biomedical Research,
        vol. 3, October, pp. 393-406.

Collen, M.F., et al., "Automated Multiphonic Screening and
1964   Diagnosis," American Journal of Public Health,
        vol. 54, May, pp. 741-750.

Colvin, F.E., "Secretaries Should Know About EDP," Hospital
1969   Topics, vol. 47, May, pp. 45-46.

Conley, D., "A Management Team Approach to Hospital Systems
1970   Analysis," Hospital Administration, Winter, pp.
        58-78.

Courtney, Sister D., "Information Processing," Hospitals,
1971   vol. 45, April 1, pp. 97-102.

Crawford, F.R., Introduction to Data Processing, Englewood
1968   Cliffs, N.J.: Prentice-Hall.

Cronkhite, L.W., Jr., "Patient Location Control as a First
1967   Step Toward A Total Information System," Hospitals
        vol. 41, May 1, pp. 107-112.

Cronkhite, L.W., Jr., "Computer Brings Order to Clinical
1969   Scheduling Systems," Hospitals, vol. 43, April
        16, pp. 55-57.

Cunningham, J.R. and J. Milan, "Radiation Treatment Planning
1970   Using a Display Oriented Small Computer," Compu-
        ters and Biomedical Research, April, pp. 159-179.

Currie, M.R., and W.P. Thompson, "Electronics in the Lab,"
1969   Hospitals, vol. 43, December 1, pp. 61-64.

Davis, L.S., et al., "Computer-Stored Medical Records,"
1968   Computers and Biomedical Research, vol. 1, May,
        pp. 452-469.

Dearden, J., "How to Organize Information Systems," Harvard
1965   Business Review, vol. 43, March-April, pp. 65-73.

Dearden, J., and R.F. Vancil, Management Control Systems:
1965   Cases and Readings, Homewood, Ill.: Richard D.
        Irwin.

DeMarco, R.M., "Planning a Computer for a Food Service De-
1968   partment," Hospitals, vol. 42, May 16, pp. 107-
        113.

DeMarco, R.M., et al., "Computer Recipes in Quantity Food
1967   Production," Hospitals, vol. 41, April 16, pp.
        88-93.

Derry, J.R., et al., "An Information System for Health
1968   Facilities Planning," American Journal of Public
        Health, vol. 58, August, pp. 1414-1421.

DeSanders, N., "Computers Basic Plans Help Doctors Initiate
1969   Rehabilitation Regimen," Modern Hospital, vol.
        113, November, pp. 97-100.

Dickson, G.W., "Management Information Decision Systems,"
1968   Business Horizons, vol. 11, December, pp. 17-26.

Dixon, R.A., "Model of a Hospital's Patient Medical Infor-
  1970   mation System," Methods of Information in Medi-
            cine, vol. 9, April, pp. 88-97.

Eilon, S., "Some Notes on Information Processing," Journal
  1968   of Management Studies, vol. 5, pp. 139-153.

Eisenberg, D.H., "Automated Patient Questionnaire Program
  1969   Measures Hospital's Effectiveness," Hospitals,
            vol. 43, September 16, pp. 66-68.

Empsey, S.L., "Computer Applications in Medicine and the
  1963   Biological Sciences: Bibliography," Communi-
            cations, ACM, vol. 6, April, p. 176.

Emrich, R., and E. Zak, "Computer Assists in Utilization
  1968   Review," Hospitals, vol. 42, August 1, pp. 56-59.

Enger, N.L., Putting Management Information Systems to Work:
  1969   Managing the Management Information Systems, N.Y.:
            American Management Association.

Engle, R.L.,Jr., "Medical Diagnosis: Present, Past, and
  1963   Future III, Diagnosis in Future, Including
            Critique on Use of Electronic Computers as
            Diagnostic Aids to Physicians," Archives of
            Internal Medicine, vol. 112, pp. 530-543.

Evans, G.W., et al., Simulation Using Digital Computers,
  1967   Englewood Cliffs, N.J.: Prentice-Hall.

Evans, M.K., and L.R. Hague, "Master Plan for Information,"
  1962   Harvard Business Review, vol. XL, January-
            February, pp. 92-103.

Feldstein, M.S., Economic Analysis for Health Service
  1968   Efficiency, Chicago, Ill.: Markham Publishing
            Co.

Filosa, L., "New Information System Uses Less Staff, Pro-
  1969   vides More Data, More Dollars," Modern Hospitals,
            vol. 112, June, pp. 87-89.

Fishburn, P.C.,"Information Analysis Without States of the
1969   World," Operations Research, vol. 17, May, pp.
        413-424.

Flack, H.F., "Electronic Data Processing and the Hospital
1967   Formulary,"   American Journal of Hospital
        Pharmacy, vol. 24, January, pp. 4-17.

Foster, J.T., "Quality of Data is First Automation Problem,"
1968   The Modern Hospital, vol. 110, April, pp.114-116.

Freed, R.N., "Get the Computer System you Want," Harvard
1969   Business Review, vol. 47, November-December, pp.
        99-108.

Gabrieli, E.R., "Computer-Orientated Documentation of Sur-
1969   gical Patients," Surgery, Gynecology, and Ob-
        stetrics, vol. 128, March, pp. 539-545.

Gabrieli, E.R., "Coordination of Medical Computing Pro-
1969   grams," Datamation, vol. 15, May, p. 117.

Gabrieli, E.R., "Prospects for Automation in the Hospital
in press   Systems," Annals of the New York Academy of
        Science.

Gabrieli, E.R., and V. Pessin, "The Computers Contribution
1966   to Information Content of Laboratory Data,"
        Journal of the American Medical Association, vol.
        198, October, pp. 63-66.

Gabrieli, E.R., et al., "Initial Experience with the Poten-
1967   tial of Data Processing and Computer Techniques
        in a Hospital Clinical Laboratory," American
        Journal of Clinical Pathology, vol. 47, January,
        pp. 60-68.

Gale, J.R., "Why Management Information Systems Fail,"
1968   Financial Executive, vol. 36, August, pp. 44-48.

Geisler, R., "THOMIS Medical Information System," Data-
1970   mation, vol. 16, June, pp. 133-136.

Gillespie, C.J., "Computerized Systems for Indexing and Re-
1971   trieving Information in Physiology Journals,"
         Physiologist, vol. 14, November, pp. 289-298.

Gillette, P.J., et al., "Hospital Information Systems,"
1970   Part I, Hospitals, vol. 44, August 16, pp. 76-
         78, Part II, vol. 44, September 1, pp. 45-48,
         110-112.

Glasser, J.H., "Health Information Systems: A Crisis or
1971   Just More of the Usual," American Journal of
         Public Health, vol. 61, August, pp. 1524-1530.

Gomberg, W., "People-Sensitive Issues for Information
1970   Systems," Wharton Quarterly, Fall, pp. 6-9.

Gordon, B.L., "Biomedical Language and Format for Manual
1968   and Computer Applications," Methods of Infor-
         mation in Medicine, vol. 7, January, pp. 5-7.

Grant, M., "Health Administration in the Computer Age,"
1969   Public Health Reports, vol. 84, May, pp. 409-414.

Greanias, E.C., "The Computer in Medicine," Datamation,
1965   vol. 11, December, pp. 25-28.

Green, F.W., "Blueprint for Shared Computer Drawn in
1969   Chicago Project," Hospitals, vol. 43, September
         1, pp. 64-69.

Greenes, R.A., et al., "Recording, Retrieval and Review
1970   of Medical Data by Physician-Computer Interac-
         tion," New England Journal of Medicine, vol.
         282, February 5, pp. 307-315.

Greenwood, F., Managing the Systems Analysis Function,
1968   N.Y.: American Management Association Press.

Greenwood, F., Guidelines to Data Processing Management,
1969   Data Processing Management Association.

Greenwood, F., and C.R. Kendrick, "Computer Technology:
1968   A Challenge for Hospital Administrators,"
         Hospital Administration, vol. 13, Summer, pp.
         62-67.

Greenwood, W.T., <u>Decision Theory and Information Systems</u>,
    1969   Cincinnati, Ohio: South-Western Publishing Co.

Grey, P.J., "Computer Aids Hospitals in Radiation Treatment
    1969   Plans," <u>Modern Hospital</u>, vol. 113, November,
            pp. 95-97.

Gue, R.L., "Mathematical Basis for Computer Planned Non-
    1969   Selective Menus," <u>Hospitals</u>, vol. 43, November
            1, pp. 102-104.

Haenszel, W.,and W.I. Lourie, Jr., "Quality Control of
    1966   Data in Large Scale Cancer Register Programs,"
            <u>Methods of Information in Medicine</u>, vol. 5, pp.
            67-74.

Haessler, H.A., "Recent Developments in Automating the
    1969   Medical History," <u>Computers and Automation</u>, vol.
            18, June 1, pp. 24-27.

Haggerty, J.R., "Computerized Information System: Accelera-
    1970   tion of Hospital Planning," <u>Hospitals</u>, vol. 44,
            November 1, pp. 43-46.

Hall, P., et al., "Data Processing System for Medical In-
    1967   formation," <u>Methods of Information in Medicine</u>,
            vol. 6, pp. 1-6.

Hammon, G.L., and S.E. Jacobs, "Shared Computer Systems--
    1970   Part 2," <u>Hospitals</u>, vol. 44, May 16, pp. 72-75.

Hart, P.F., "Computer Applications in Hospitals--A Look
    1966   Ahead," <u>Canadian Hospital</u>, vol. 43, January,
            pp. 40-43.

Hartman, W.M., <u>Information Systems Handbook: Analysis,</u>
    1969   <u>Requirements, Determination, Design and Develop-</u>
            <u>ment, Implementation and Evaluation</u>, N.Y.:
            McGraw-Hill.

Hayes, J.E., Jr., "Medical Information System of 1975,"
    1970   <u>Computers and Biomedical Research</u>, vol. 3,
            October, pp. 555-560.

Hechinger, S., and B. Vick, "Computer Scheduling Helps Con-
1968   trol Maintenance Work," The Modern Hospital, vol.
110, May, pp. 160-161.

Heller, W.M., "Data Processing in Drug Distribution Sys-
1968   tems," Hospitals, vol. 42, December 1, pp. 73-78.

Hennessey, T.F., "EDP and the Small Hospital," Hospitals,
1970   vol. 44, February 16, pp. 61-63.

Heyel, C., Computers, Office Machines and the New Infor-
1969   mation Technology, N.Y.: Macmillan.

Hicks, G.P., et al., "Routine Use of Small Digital Compu-
1966   ters in Clinical Laboratory," Journal of the
American Medical Association, vol. 196, June
13, pp. 973-978.

Hinnicks, J.R., "The Computer in Manpower Research,"
1970   Personnel Administration, March-April, pp. 37-44.

Hofmann, P.B., and G.O. Barnett, "Time Sharing Increases
1968   Benefits of Computer Use," Hospitals, vol. 42,
June 16, pp. 62-67.

Hofmann, P.B., et al., "Computers: Great Future, Perilous
1968   Present," Modern Hospitals, vol. 111, July,
pp. 99-100, 148.

Hofmann, P.B., et al., "Automated Patient Census Operation:
1969   Design, Development, Evaluation, Massachusetts
General Hospital," Hospital Topics, vol. 47,
May, pp. 39-41.

Hodges, T.H., and S.I. Allen, "Data Processing System
1968   Supplies Intravenous Additive Information,"
Hospitals, vol. 42, November 16, pp. 103-105.

Holmes, R.W., "Information Systems Review for Senior Manage-
1969   ment," Financial Executive, vol. 37, April, pp.
56-62.

Homer, E., "A Generalized Model for Analyzing Management
1962   Information Systems," Management Science, vol.
8, July, pp. 500-515.

"Hospitals Share Computer to Aid Patient Service," Systems,
    1966   June, pp. 12-14, 30, 39.

Howell, J.P., "Annual Administrative Reviews, Data Process-
    1970   ing," Hospitals, vol. 44, April 1, pp. 60-66.

Huff, W.S., Jr., "Shared Computer Time: Big Benefits for
    1969   Small Hospital," Modern Hospital, vol. 113,
            November, pp. 88-91, 154.

Jackson, J.T., "Information Systems for Management Planning"
    1962   Data Processing, vol. 4, March, pp. 25-27.

Jacobs, H., "Natural Language Information Retrieval Sys-
    1968   tem," Methods of Information in Medicine, vol.
            7, pp. 8-10.

Jacobus, G.C., "Sorting Sense from Nonsense in Hospital
    1968   ADP Programs," Hospitals, vol. 42, June 16,
            pp. 62-67.

James, G.J., "Planning a Communication-Based Management
    1964   Information System," Computers and Automation,
            vol. 13, October, pp. 20-21.

Jydstrup, R., and M.J. Gross, "Cost of Information Handling
    1966   in Hospitals," Health Services Research, vol.
            1, Winter, pp. 239-271.

Kanon, D., "Computer Analyzes Lab Tests, Does Own Quality
    1969   Control," Modern Hospital, vol. 113, November,
            pp. 105-107.

Kanon, D., and Sister C. Bilsborough, "Patient Information
    1969   Utilizes Central Dictation," Hospitals, vol.
            43, October 1, pp. 56-59.

Kavet, J., and J.D. Thompson, "Computers Can Tell you What
    1967   Will Happen Before it Happens," The Modern
            Hospital, vol. 109, December, pp. 102-105.

Keller, T.F., "The Hospital Information System," Hospital.
    1969   Administration, vol. 14, Winter, pp. 40-50.

Kelly, J.F., Computerized Management Information Systems,
1970 N.Y.: Macmillan.

Kelly, R.C., "Computerized Hospital Information System: A
1970 Control Mechanism," Hospital Progress, vol. 51,
April, pp. 42-46.

Kemeny, J.G., and T.E. Kurtz, "Dartmouth Time Sharing,"
1968 Science, vol. 162, October 11, pp. 223-228.

Kleinmuntz, B., Clinical Information Processing by Computer,
1969 N.Y.: Holt, Rinehart & Winston.

Kolouch, F.T., "Computer Shows How Patient Stays Vary,"
1965 Modern Hospital, vol. 105, November, pp. 130-134.

Korein, J., et al., "Computer Processing of Medical Data by
1966 Variable Field-Length Format, III, Statistical
Analysis of Narrative Content," Journal of the
American Medical Association, vol. 196, June 13,
pp. 957-963.

Kosty, E.W., "Centralizing Data Processing in a Two Loca-
1968 tion Hospital," Management Services, vol. 5,
November-December, pp. 51-54.

Krauss, L.I., Computer-Based Management Information Systems,
1970 N.Y.: American Management Association Press.

Krismer, J.R., "Comprehensive Health Operating and Infor-
1971 mation Systems," Transactions of the American
Academy of Ophthalmology and Otolaryngology,
vol. 75, September-October, pp. 1126-1131.

Laden, H.N., and T.R. Gildersleeve, Systems Design for
1963 Computer Application, N.Y.: John Wiley & Sons.

Lamott, K., "Using Computers in Planning and Programming,"
1967 Hospitals, vol. 41, May 1, pp. 127-130.

Lamson, B.G., et al., "Hospital-Wide System for Handling
1967 Medical Data," Hospitals, vol. 41, May 1,
pp. 67-80.

Lande, H., How to Use the Computer in Business Planning,
1969   Englewood Cliffs, N.J.: Prentice-Hall.

Last, J.M., "Primary Medical Care 1. Record Keeping,"
1965   Milbank Memorial Fund Quarterly, vol. 43, April,
pp. 266-276.

LaValle, J.M., and A. Rappaport, "On the Economics of Ac-
1968   quiring Information of Imperfect Reliability,"
Accounting Review, vol. 43, April, pp. 225-230.

Ledley, R.S., "The Use of Electronic Computers in Medical
1960   Data Processing Aids in Diagnosis, Current Information Retrieval and Medical Research Keeping,"
IRE Trans. on Medical Electronics, vol. 7,
January, pp. 31-47.

Ledley, R.S., Use of Computers in Biology and Medicine,
1965   N.Y.: McGraw-Hill, pp. 451-464.

Ledley, R.S., "Digital Electronic Computers in Biomedical
1969   Science," Science, vol. 130, November 6, pp.
1225-1235.

Ledley, R.S., and L.B. Lusted, "Reasoning Foundations of
1959   Medical Diagnosis," Science, vol. 130, July
3, pp. 9-21.

Ledley, R.S., and L.B. Lusted, "Computers in Medical Data
1960   Processing," Operations Research, May-June, pp.
299-310.

Leighton, E., and P. Headly, "Computer Analysis of Length
1968   of Stay," Hospital Progress, vol. 49, April,
pp. 67-70.

Levy, R.P., and M.R. Cammarn, "Information Systems Appli-
1968   cations in Medicine," Annual Review of Information Science Technology, vol. 3, pp. 397-428.

Levy, R.P., et al., "Computer Handling of Ambulatory
1964   Clinic Records," Journal of the American Medical
Association, vol. 190, December 21, pp. 1033-1037.

Lindberg, D.A., "Collection, Evaluation and Transmission
   1967   of Hospital Laboratory Data," Methods of Infor-
          mation in Medicine, vol. 6, July, pp. 97-107.

Lindberg, D.A., The Computer and Medical Care, Springfield,
   1968   Ill.: Charles C Thomas.

Lindberg, D.A., et al., "Computer Sets Stage for Multi-
   1967   Testing," Modern Hospital, vol. 108, April,
          pp. 128-130.

Lodwick, G.S., et al., "Computer Diagnosis of Primary Bone
   1963   Tumors, Preliminary Report," Radiology, vol.
          80, January-June, pp. 273-275.

MacDonald, L.K., "Computerized Test Measurements," Hospi-
   1961   tals, vol. 35, February 16, pp. 72-75.

Madden, E.E., Jr., and R.H. Dreyfus, "Outpatient Pharmacy
   1968   Prescription Automation," American Journal of
          Hospital Pharmacy, vol. 25, January, pp. 20-25.

Marschak, J., "Economics of Inquiring, Communicating, and
   1968   Deciding," American Economic Review, vol. 58,
          May, pp. 1-19.

Martin, F.F., Computer Modeling and Simulation, N.Y.: John
   1968   Wiley & Sons.

Mathews, M.V., "Choosing a Scientific Computer for Service,"
   1968   Science, vol. 161, July 5, pp. 23-27.

Mayne, J.G., "Experience with the Use of Automation for
   1969   Collecting and Recording Medicine History Data,"
          Methods of Information in Medicine, vol. 8,
          April, pp. 53-59.

Mayne, J.G., et al., "Towards Automating Medical History,"
   1968   Mayo Clinic Proceedings, vol. 43, pp. 1-25.

McCarn, D., and D. Moriarity, "Computers in Medicine,"
   1971   Hospitals, vol. 45, January 1, pp. 37-39.

McCosh, A., "Computerized Cost Finding Systems," Hospital
   1969   Financial Management, vol. 23, November, pp. 18-22.

Melrose, P., "Automated Medication Order System," <u>Hospi-</u>
1970   <u>tals</u>, vol. 44, September 16, pp. 66-73.

Meyer, E., "Electronic Data Processing Benefits Both Buyer
1967   and Seller," <u>Hospital Management</u>, vol. 103,
        June, pp. 107-108.

<u>Modern Hospital</u>, "Computer Helps Cardiologist by Converting
1969   ECG Signals into Digits for Analysis," vol.
        113, November, pp. 91-93.

Monagle, W.J., and T.D. LaSalle, "Computerized Multiphasic
1969   Screening: More Tests, More Speed--But Not More
        Cost," <u>Modern Hospital</u>, vol. 113, November,
        pp. 100-103.

Moon, J.E., "Computerized Pharmacy Systems Solves Hospitals
1969   Drug Inventory Problems," <u>Modern Hospital</u>, vol.
        113, November, pp. 118-124.

Moon, J.E., "On Line Computer System is Memory for Patient
1969   Care Data," <u>Modern Hospital</u>, vol. 113, July,
        pp. 70-72.

Moore, F.J., "Information Technologies and Health Care,"
1970   <u>Archives of Internal Medicine</u>, vol. 125, January,
        pp. 157-161; February, pp. 351-355; March, pp.
        503-508; April, pp. 711-715.

Needles, B., Jr., "An Internal Control Plan for a Hospital
1969   Computer Center," <u>Hospital Financial Management</u>,
        vol. 23, October, pp. 15-18.

<u>New York Academy of Science, Annals of</u>, "Conference on the
1968   Use of Data Mechanization and Computers in Clini-
        cal Medicine, Sessions on the Hospital as a
        Cybernetic System and Prospects for Automation in
        ꞌ   Hospital System," vol. 30, January, p. 627.

<u>New York Academy of Science, Annals of</u>, "The Use of Data
1969   Mechanization and Computers in Clinical Medi
        cine," vol. 161, September 30, pp. 371-830.

Noble, J.H., Jr., "Designing Information Systems for Com-
1970   prehensive Health Planning," Inquiry, vol. 7,
        pp. 34-40.

Norton, J.H., "Information Systems: Some Basic Considera-
1969   tions," Management Review, vol. 58, September,
        p. 2.

Oliver, J.A., "Electronic Data Processing," Hospitals,
1970   vol. 44, June 1, pp. 72-77.

Omlor, J.J., "Management Information System for Planning,
1970   Forecasting and Budgeting," Management Account-
        ing, vol. 51, March, pp. 13-16.

Osborn, J.J., and J.O. Beaumont, "Computerized Intensive
1970   Care," Hospitals, vol. 44, June 16, pp. 40-53.

Pastena, L., The Possibility of Using Electronic Processors
1967   in Psychiatry, Rome: University of Rome.

Polissar, J., "Hospital Computer Applications: Possible
1969   and Projected," Hospital Topics, vol. 47, April,
        pp. 40-41.

Potter, B., "Doctor-Computer Dialogue Speeds Orders," The
1967   Modern Hospital, vol. 109, July, p. 10.

Potter, B., "Computer Clerk is Key to This System," The
1968   Modern Hospital, vol. 110, April, pp. 111-113.

Powers, A.M., and G.F. Whitlock, Jr., "Computerized Employee
1968   Data Aid Administrative Decision-Making,"
        Hospitals, vol. 42, August 1, pp. 60-63.

Pratt, A.W., and L.B. Thomas, "Information Processing
1966   System for Pathology Data," Pathology Annual,
        1966 Series, editor: S.C. Sommers, N.Y.:
        Appleton-Century-Crofts.

Pribor, H.C., et al., "Small Computers Do Big Job in This
1968   Hospital Laboratory," Modern Hospital, vol.
        110, April, pp. 104-107.

Provost, G.P., "History and Status of the ASHP Drug Coding
  1968   and Listing Services," American Journal of Hos-
          pital Pharmacy, vol. 25, January, pp. 12, 19.

Race, D., and E.R. Gabrieli, "Probability Prediction System
  1967   Applied to a Hospital Transfusion System," in
          Automation in Analytical Chemistry, N.Y.:
          Mediad, Inc.

Rappaport, A.   (ed.), Information for Decision Making:
  1970   Quantitative and Behavioral Dimensions, Engle-
          wood Cliffs, N.J.: Prentice-Hall.

Rappoport, A.E., and W.B. Gennaro, "You Get the Blood,
  1969   Computer Does CBC," Modern Hospital, vol. 113,
          November, pp. 103-105.

Rappoport, A.E., and W.B. Gennaro, and W.J. Constandse,
  1968   "Computer Laboratory Link is Base of Hospital
          Information System," Modern Hospital, vol. 1]0,
          April, pp. 94-102.

Rappoport, A.E., and E.N. Rappoport, "Laboratory Automation"
  1970   Hospitals, vol. 44, August 16, pp. 114-121.

Reading, G., and H.W. Hale, Jr., Computer Oriented Docu-
  in press mentation of the Surgical Patient.

Reed, R., Jr., and W.E. Stanley, "Optimizing Control of
  1965   Hospital Inventories," The Journal of Industrial
          Engineering, vol. 16, January-February, pp. 48-51.

Reeves, P.N., "Taming the Tiger: How to Make Your EDP
  1969   Systems Pay Off," Hospital Topics, vol. 47,
          April, pp. 36-39.

Reilly, N.B., "Computers in Medicine," Datamation, vol.
  1969   15, May, pp. 46-49.

Rikli, A.E., et al., "Study Suggests Value of Shared Compu-
  1966   ters," Modern Hospital, vol. 106, May, pp.
          100-108.

Rikli, A.E., and S.I.Allen, "The Federal Survey Examines
1968   Computerized Admission Systems," The Modern Hos-
        pital, vol. 111, October, pp. 99-102.

Roberto, E.A., "A Case for the Computer in the Small Hospi-
1969   tal," Hospital Topics, vol. 47, May, pp. 33-39.

Rosenbaum, C.P., "Computer Simplifies Record Keeping and
1968   Review in Psychiatric Clinic," Hospitals, vol.
        42, April 16, pp. 70-73.

Rosner, M.W., "Economic Determinants of Organizational
1968   Innovation," Administrative Science Quarterly,
        vol. 12, March, pp. 614-625.

Ross, J.E., Management by Information System, Englewood
1970   Cliffs, N.J.: Prentice-Hall.

Rowe, A.J., "Coming to Terms with Computer Management
1968   Systems," Financial Executive, vol. 36, April,
        pp. 64-73.

Runck, H.M., "Computer Planning for Hospitals: The Large-
1969   Scale Education and Involvement of Employees,"
        Computers and Automation, vol. 18, June 1, pp.
        33-35.

Russell, J.A., "Small Computers--Bridge to Total Systems,"
1968   Hospitals, vol. 42, October 1, pp. 62+.

Sager, J.F., "Recipe and Ingredient Control by Computer,"
1969   Hospitals, vol. 43, September 16, pp. 87-89.

Sanazaro, P.J., "Automatic Multiphasic Health Testing,"
1971   Hospitals, vol. 45, March 1, pp. 41-43.

Sanders, D.H., Computers and Management, N.Y. McGraw-Hill.
1970

Sanders, M.G., "The Computer and Total Medical Information
1969   Processing," Canadian Hospital, vol. 46, Octo-
        ber, pp. 64-69.

Scadding, J.G., "Diagnosis: The Clinician and the Computer",
1967   Lancet, vol. 2, October 21, pp. 877-882.

Schneider, J.H., "Selective Dissemination and Indexing of
1971   Scientific Information," <u>Science</u>, vol. 173,
        July 23, pp. 300-308.

Schwartz, M.D., "Status of Hospital Information Systems,"
1970   <u>Hospital Progress</u>, vol. 51, June 6, pp. 52-60.

Seibert,S., "Utilization of Computer Equipment and Tech-
1967   niques in Prescription Process at Los Angeles
        County General Hospital," <u>Drug Intelligence and
        Clinical Pharmacy</u>, vol. 1, November, pp. 342-350.

Sherman, S.R., et al., "Computer Intervention with People,
1970   Patients, and Physicians," <u>Medical Care</u>, vol. 8,
        July-August, pp. 276-286.

Siker, E., et al., "The New Haven Health Information
1971   System: A Model for Relating Health and Census
        Data," <u>Inquiry</u>, vol. 8, December, pp. 58-62.

Siler, W., and H. Korn, "Working Total Information System
1967   is at Least Year Away," <u>Hospitals</u>, vol. 41,
        May 1, pp. 99-104.

Slack, W., "Computer Based Interviewing," <u>Science</u>, vol.
1971   171, January 8, pp. 84-87.

Slack, W.V., et al., "Computer Based Medical History
1966   Systems," <u>New England Journal of Medicine</u>, vol.
        274, January 27, pp. 194-198.

Slack, W.V., et al., "Computer Based Physical Examination
1967   System," <u>Journal of the American Medical Associ-
        ation</u>, vol. 200, April 17, pp. 224-228.

Slee, V.N., "Information Systems and Measurement Tools,"
1966   <u>Journal of the American Medical Association</u>,
        vol. 196, June 20, pp. 1063-1065.

Smalley, E.H., "An Inservice Approach to Management Systems
1967   Improvement," <u>Hospitals</u>, vol. 41, July 1, p. 63.

Smith, J.L., "The Computer, Its Impact on the Physician,
1969   the Muse and the Administrator," <u>Hospitals</u>, vol.
        43, September 16, pp. 61-65.

Smith, P.T., Computers, Systems, and Profits, N.Y.: Ameri-
1969   can Management Association Press.

Smith, R.M., "How to Automate a Hospital," Management Ser-
1966   vices, vol. 3, July-August, pp. 48-53.

Souder, J.J., "Computers Can Bring a New Rationality Into
1968   Hospital Design," The Modern Hospital, vol. 110,
        March, pp. 80-86.

Spivey B., and J. O'Neill, "The Use of Optical Scanning as
1969   a Means of Computer Impact in Medicine," Journal
        of the American Medical Association, vol. 208,
        April 28, pp. 665-672.

Starr, M.K., Systems Management of Operations, Englewood
1971   Cliffs, N.J.: Prentice-Hall.

Steffy, D.E., et al., "Emergency Room Information System
1968   Speeds Collections," The Modern Hospital, vol.
        110, April, pp. 68-69.

Sterling, T.D., et al., "Is Medical Diagnosis General
1966   Computer Problem?" Journal of the American Medi-
        cal Association, vol. 198, October 17, pp. 281-
        286.

Stokes, J., III, and R.M. Hayes, "Commentary on the Bio-
1970   medical Information System," Journal of Medical
        Education, vol. 45, April, pp. 243-249.

Straumfjord, J.V., Jr., et al., "Electronic Data Processing
1967   System for Clinical Laboratory: System Used for
        All Laboratory Sections," Technical Bulletin of
        The Registry of Medical Technologists, vol. 37,
        April, pp. 91-106.

Summers, H., "The Computer in the Hospital Laboratory: Is
1970   it Premature?" International Journal of Bio-
        medical Computing, January 1, pp. 31-39.

Templeton, A.W., et al., "Radiate: New Concept of Computer
1965   Coding, Transmitting, Storing and Retrieving
        Radiological Data," Radiology, vol. 85, pp.
        811-817.

Thoren, B.J., et al., "Attitude Study, Training Helps Em-
1969   ployees Adapt to Use of Computers," Hospitals,
        vol. 43, March, pp. 61-64.

Thurlow, R.M., "More Legal Risks with Computer Medicine,"
1969   Medical Economics, vol. 46, March 3, p. 126.

Tomeski, E.A., The Computer Revolution: The Executive and
1969   the New Information Technology, N.Y.: Macmillan.

Toronto, A.F., et al., "Evaluation of Computer Program for
1963   Diagnosis of Congenital Heart Disease," Progress
        in Cardiovascular Diseases, vol. 5, no. 4, pp.
        362-377.

Travis, J.W., "Computers, Patient Care and Medical Educa-
1969   tion," New Physician, vol. 18, August, pp. 629-
        633.

United States Air Force, Guide for Auditing Automatic Data
1966   Processing, Washington, D.C.; Government Printing
        Office.

Vallbona, C., "Preparing Medical Record Data for Computer
1967   Processing," Hospitals, vol. 41, May 1, pp. 113-
        118.

Vallbona, C., et al., "Experience with On-line Monitoring
1966   in Critical Illness," I.E.E.E. Spectrum, vol.
        3, pp. 136-140.

VanHoudnos, H.M., "Automated Data System: How it Aids
1971   Mental Hospital's Staff," Medical Record News,
        vol. 42, August, pp. 26-31.

Vermillon, C.O., "Data Processing Methods," Hospitals,
1968   vol. 42, April 1, pp. 37-40.

Walker, D.E., Information System Science and Technology,
1967   Washington, D.C.: Thompson Book Co.

Wartak, J., Computers in Electrocardiography, Springfield,
1970   Ill.: Charles C Thomas.

Wefsey, M.M., Management of Automatic Data Processing Sys-
    1968   tems, Washington, D.C.: Thompson Book Co.

Weil, M.H., et al., "Experience with Digital Computer for
    1966   Study and Improved Management of Critically Ill,"
            Journal of the American Medical Association, vol.
            198, November 28, pp. 1011-1016.

Weil, T.P., "80 Basic Applications for ADP Equipment,"
    1967   Hospitals, vol. 41, May 1, pp. 81-89.

Weisbrod, B.A., "Some Problems of Pricing and Resource Al-
    1965   location in a Non-Profit Industry - The Hospi-
            tals," The Journal of Business, vol. 38, January,
            pp. 18-28.

Wessel, M.R., "Problems of Liability for the E.D.P. Services
    1970   Industry," Computers and Automation, vol. 19,
            September, pp. 18-21.

White, W.L., "Low Cost Laboratory Reporting System Uses
    1969   Business Computers," Hospitals, vol. 43, July 16,
            pp. 83-86.

Wiener, N., "Some Moral and Technical Consequences of Auto-
    1960   mation," Science, vol. 131, May, pp. 1355-1358.

Wilber, S.A., and W.S. Derrick, "Patient Monitoring and
    1965   Anesthetic Management: Physiological Communica-
            tions Network," Journal of the American Medical
            Association, vol. 191, March 15, pp. 893-898.

Williams, G.Z., "Use of Data Processing and Automation in
    1964   Clinical Pathology," Military Medicine, vol. 129,
            June, pp. 502-509.

Williams, T.H., and C.H. Griffin, Management Information:
    1967   A Quantitative Accent, Homewood, Ill.: Richard
            D. Irwin.

Wilson, H., "Automated Data Processing in a Modern Hos-
    1962   pital," U.S.G.R.R., No. PB-166461.

Wood, C.T., and A. LaMontagne, "A Computer Assists Advance
     1969   Bed Bookings," Hospitals, vol. 43, March 1,
               pp. 67-69.

Yoder, R.D., "Preparing Medical Record Data for Computer
     1966   Processing," Hospitals, vol. 40, August 16, pp.
               75-85.

Youngquist, C.R., "Computer Speeds Reporting of Laboratory
     1968   Test Results," Hospitals, vol. 42, January 1,
               pp. 37+.

Zannetos, Z.S., "Towards Intelligent Management Information
     1968   Systems," Industrial Management Review, vol. 9,
               Spring, pp. 21-38.

Part 9.

EVALUATION

Anderson, A.J., and I. Altman, Methodology in Evaluating
    1962   the Quality of Medical Care, An Annotated Selected
            Bibliography 1955-1961, Pittsburgh, Pa.;   Univer-
            sity of Pittsburgh Press.

Bailey, M.C., "Evaluation of Public Health Nursing Services
    1969   Through a Study of Patient Progress," in H.C.
            Schulberg, A. Sheldon, and F. Baker (eds.), Pro-
            gram Evaluation in the Health Fields, N.Y.:
            Behavioral Publications.

Bellin, L.E., "Medical Audit: Bitter Pill Is Here and Now,"
    1971   Medical Opinion, vol. 7, December, pp. 22-26.

Borgatta, E., "Research Problems in Evaluation of Health
    1966   Service Demonostrations," Milbank Memorial Fund
            Quarterly, vol. 44, pp. 182-201.

Deniston, O.L., and I.M. Rosenstock, "Evaluating Health
    1970   Programs," Public Health Report, vol. 85,
            September, pp. 835-840.

Densen, P.M., et al., "Research, Program Planning and Evalu-
    1966   ation," Public Health Reports, vol. 81, January,
            pp. 49-56.

Donabedian, A., "Evaluating the Quality of Medical Care,"
    1969   in H.C. Schulberg, A. Sheldon, and F. Baker
            (eds.), Program Evaluation in the Health Fields,
            N.Y.: Behavioral Publications.

Ellis, E.F., "Evaluation of National Health Programs: A
    1971   Disparity Between Desire and Practice in Local
            Health Departments," American Journal of Public
            Health, vol. 61, September, pp. 1826-1831.

Flagle, C.D., "Evaluation Techniques for Medical Information
    1970   Systems," Computers and Biomedical Research,
            vol. 3, October, pp. 407-414.

Gordis, L., and M. Markowitz, "Evaluation of Comprehensive
1971   and Continuous Pediatric Care," Pediatrics, vol.
48, November, pp. 766-777.

Gordon, D.W., "Problems in the Measurement and Evaluation
1971   of Patient Systems and Behavior," Medical Care,
vol. 9, September-October, pp. 396-404.

Harper, D., and H. Babigian, "Evaluation Research: The
1971   Consequences of Program Evaluation," Mental
Hygiene, vol. 55, April, pp. 151-156.

Hilleboe, H.E., and M. Schaefer, "Evaluation in Community
1968   Health: Relating Results to Goals," Bulletin
of the New York Academy of Medicine, 2nd series,
vol. 44, no. 2, pp. 140-158.

Kish, A.I., "Adapting Health Manpower to Consumer Needs
1971   and Cultural Expectations," Inquiry, vol. 8,
September, pp. 39-50.

Klein, S.F., "Toward a Framework for Evaluating Health
1971   Education Activities of a Family Planning
Program," American Journal of Public Health,
vol. 61, June, pp. 1096-1109.

Last, J.M., "Evaluation of Medical Care," The Medical Jour-
1965   nal of Australia, November 6, pp. 781-785.

Levy, L.,   "An Evaluation of a Mental Health
1971   Program by Use of Selected Operating Statistics,"
American Journal of Public Health, vol. 61,
October, pp. 2038-2045.

Lincoln, T.L., and G.H. Weiss,"A Statistical Evaluation of
1964   Recurrent Medical Examinations," Operations
Research, vol. 12, March-April, pp. 187-205.

Litsios, S., "The Principles and Methods of Evaluation of
1971   National Health Plans," International Journal of
Health Services, vol. 1, February, pp. 79-85.

McCaffree, K.M., "The Cost of Mental Health Care Under
  1969   Changing Treatment Methods," in H.C. Schulberg,
          A. Sheldon, and F. Baker (eds.), <u>Program Evalua-
          tion in the Health Fields</u>, N.Y.: Behavioral
          Publications.

Monk, M., et al., "Evaluation of an Anti-Smoking Program
  1969   Among High School Students," in H.C. Schulberg,
          A. Sheldon, and F. Baker (eds.), <u>Program Evalua-
          tion in the Health Fields</u>, N.Y.: Behavioral
          Publications.

Morehead, M.A., "Evaluating Quality of Medical Care in the
  1970   Neighborhood Health Center Program of the Office
          of Economic Opportunity," <u>Medical Care</u>, vol. 8,
          March-April, pp. 118-131.

Morehead, M.A., et al., <u>A Study of the Quality of Hospital
  1964   Care Secured by a Sample of Teamster Family Mem-
          bers in New York City</u>, N.Y.: Columbia University,
          School of Public Health and Administrative
          Medicine.

Peterson, O.L., "Evaluation of the Quality of Medical Care,"
  1963   <u>New England Journal of Medicine</u>, vol. 269, pp.
          1238-1245.

Reiffen, B., <u>Medical Care Evaluation and Systems Analysis</u>,
  1970   Document No. PB-200 253, Springfield, Va.:
          National Technical Information Service.

Richart, R.H., "Evaluation of a Medical Data System,"
  1970   <u>Computers and Biomedical Research</u>, vol. 3, Octo-
          ber, pp. 415-425.

Rifka, G., and Y. Khoury, "Preliminary Evaluation of a
  1971   School of Public Health Through its Physician
          Graduates: American University at Beirut,"
          <u>American Journal of Public Health</u>, vol. 61, Nov-
          ember, pp. 2290-2293.

Roemer, M.I., "Evaluation of Health Service Programs and
  1971   Levels of Measurement," <u>HSMHA Health Reports</u>,
          vol. 86, September, pp. 839-848.

Schulberg, H.C., and F. Baker, "Program Evaluation in Models
   1969   and the Implementation of Research Findings," in
            H.C. Schulberg, A. Sheldon, and F. Baker (eds.),
            Program Evaluation in the Health Fields, N.Y.:
            Behavioral Publications.

Slee, V.N., "How to Know if You Have Quality Control," Hos-
   1972   pital Progress, vol. 53, January, pp. 38-43.

Stitzel, P.J., "Evaluation of the Hospital Accreditation
   1971   Program of American Osteopathic Association,"
            Osteopathic Hospital, vol. 15, November, pp. 5-9.

Suchman, E., Evaluative Research, Principles and Practice
   1967   in Public Service and Social Action Programs, N.Y.:
            Russell Sage Foundation.

Tripodi, T., et al., "Dilemmas in Evaluation: Implications
   1970   for Administrators of Social Action Programs,"
            American Journal of Orthopsychiatry, vol. 40,
            October, pp. 850-857.

White, K.L., "Primary Medical Care for Families--Organiza-
   1967   tion and Evaluation," New England Journal of
            Medicine, vol. 277, pp. 847-852.

Williamson, J.W., "Evaluating Quality of Patient Care,"
   1971   Journal of the American Medical Association, vol.
            218, October, pp. 564-569.

Yordy, K.D., "Evaluation of National Health Programs: On
   1971   The Federal Level," American Journal of Public
            Health, vol. 61, September, pp. 1803-1808.

Part 10.

CONTROL

Bell, G.D., "Determinants of Span of Control," _American_
1967   _Journal of Sociology_, vol. 73, July, pp. 100-109.

Berger, J., et al., "Evaluations and the Formation and
1969   Maintenance of Performance Expectations," _Human_
        Relations, vol. December, pp. 481-502.

Berkurtt, G.J., "Behavioral Science: Is the Cure Worth
1970   It?" _Dun's_, vol. 95, May, pp. 38-41.

Berne, E., _Games People Play_, N.Y.: Franklin Watts.

Blau, P.M., _Exchange and Power in Social Life_, N.Y.: John
1964   Wiley & Sons.

Bonjean, C.M., and M.D. Grimes, "Bureaucracy and Alienation:
1970   A Dimensional Approach," _Social Forces_, vol.
        48, March, pp. 365-373.

Bonjean, C.M., and G.G. Vance, "A Short-Form Measure of
1968   Self-Actualization," _Journal of Applied Behav-_
        ioral Science, vol. 4, July-August-September,
        pp. 299-312.

Braunstein, D.N., "Interpersonal Behavior in a Changing
1970   Organization," _Journal of Applied Psychology_,
        vol. 54, April, pp. 184-191.

Chorba, R.W., and J.L. Sanders, "Planning Models for Tuber-
1971   culosis Control," _Health Services Research_,
        vol. 6, Summer, pp. 144-167.

Clark, J.V., "Task Group Theory: (I) Goals and the Client
1970   System; (II) Intervention and Problems of Prac-
        tice," _Human Relations_, vol. 23, August, pp.
        263-277; October, pp. 383-403.

Denhardt, R.B., "Leadership Style, Worker Involvement, and
1970   Deference to Authority," _Sociology and Social_
        Research, vol. 54, January, pp. 172-180.

Dyer, W.G., "Congruence and Control," Journal of Applied
   1969   Behavioral Science, vol. 5, no. 2, pp. 161-173.

Ericson, R.F., "Organizational Cybernetics and Human Values,"
   1970   Academy of Management Journal, vol. 13, March,
           pp. 49-66.

Evans, M.G., "The Effects of Supervisory Behavior on the
   1970   Path-Goal Relationship," Organizational Behavior
           and Human Performance, vol. 5, May, pp. 277-298.

Feldstein, M.S., "Developments in Health Service Adminis-
   1963   tration and Financial Control," Medical Care,
           vol. 3, July-September, pp. 171-177.

Feldstein, M.S., "Hospital Cost Inflation: Study of Non-
   1971   profit Price Dynamics," American Economic Review,
           vol. 61, December, pp. 853-872.

Friedlander, F., "The Primacy of Trust as a Facilitator of
   1970   Further Group Accomplishment," Journal of Ap-
           plied Behavioral Science, vol. 6, no. 4, pp.
           387-400.

Ginzberg, E., "Hospital Costs: Sense and Nonsense," Rhode
   1971   Island Medical Journal, vol. 54, August, pp.
           409-412.

Grotnes, M.S., Establishment of a Forms Control System in
   1970   an Acute Care General Hospital, Cincinnati, Ohio:
           Xavier University, May 15.

Haire, M., "The Concept of Power and the Concept of Man,"
   1962   in G. Strother (ed.), Social Science Approaches
           to Business Behavior, Homewood, Ill.: Dorsey
           Press.

Hammerton, J.G., "Management and Motivation," California
   1970   Management Review, vol. 13, Winter, pp. 51-56.

Hofstede, G.H., The Game of Budget Control, Assen, The
   1967   Netherlands: Van Gorcum & Co.

House, R.J., and J.B. Miner, "Merging Management and Be-
1969   havioral Theory: The Interaction Between Span of
        Control and Group Size," Administrative Science
        Quarterly, vol. 14, September, pp. 451-464.

Katz, D., "The Motivational Basis of Organizational Be-
1964   havior," Behavioral Science, vol. 9, April,
        pp. 131-146.

Kolb, D.A., and R.E. Boyatzis, "Goal-Setting and Self-
1970   Directed Behavior Change," Human Relations, vol.
        23, October, pp. 439-457.

Kolb, D.A., and R.E. Boyatzis, "On the Dynamics of the
1970   Helping Relationship," Journal of Applied Be-
        havioral Science, vol. 6, no. 3, pp. 267-288.

Korman, A.K., "Toward an Hypothesis of Work Behavior,"
1970   Journal of Applied Psychology, vol. 54, Part 1,
        February, pp. 31-41.

Kunkel, J.H., "Some Behavioral Aspects of the Ecological
1967   Approach to Social Organization," American
        Journal of Sociology, vol. 73, July, pp. 12-29.

Lawler, E.E., III., "Job Attitudes and Employee Motiva-
1970   tion: Theory, Research, and Practice," Per-
        sonnel Psychology, vol. 23, Summer, pp. 223-237.

Locke, E.A., "What is Job Satisfaction?" Organizational
1969   Behavior and Human Performance, vol. 4, November,
        pp. 309-336.

Locke, E.A., "Job Satisfaction and Job Performance: A
1970   Theoretical Analysis," Organizational Behavior
        and Human Performance, vol. 5, September, pp.
        484-500.

London, P., Behavior Control, N.Y.: Harper & Row.
1969

Ludwig, P.E., "Dollars and Sense," W.K. Kellogg Foundation.
1971

MacDonald, G.E., "Cost Control: The Physician's Role,"
    1971   Hospitals, vol. 45, April 16, pp. 55-59.

Mathews, C.L., "Systematic Monitoring of Costs," Hospitals,
    1971   vol. 45, December 16, pp. 77-82.

Megley, J.E., III., "Management and the Behavioral Sciences:
    1970   Theory Z," Personnel Journal, vol. 49, March,
            pp. 216-221.

Meyer, M.W., "Expertness and the Span of Control," American
    1968   Sociological Review, vol. 33, December, pp. 944-
            951.

Migliore, R. H., "Improving Worker Productivity Through
    1970   Communicating Knowledge of Work Results,"
            Management of Personnel Quarterly, vol. 9, Summer,
            pp. 26-32.

Miles, R.E., "Human Relations or Human Resources?" Harvard
    1965   Business Review, vol. 43, pp. 148-154.

Miljus, R.C., "Effective Leadership and the Motivation of
    1970   Human Resources," Personnel Journal, vol. 49,
            pp. 36-40.

Nagy, E.J., and G.E. Moore, Nurse Quality Control Study,
    1971   Denver, Colo.: Midtown Hospital Association.

Pearsall, M., and S.M. Kern, "Behavioral Science, Nursing
    1967   Services and the Collaborative Process; A Case
            Study," Journal of Applied Behavioral Science,
            vol. 3, pp. 243-266.

Pugh, D.S., "Organization Behavior: An Approach from
    1969   Psychology," Human Relations, vol. 22, pp. 345-
            354.

Reginald, Sister M., Internal Control, Cincinnati, Ohio:
    1970   Xavier University Press, May.

Rice, D.P., "Measurement and Application of Illness Costs,"
    1969   Public Health Reports, vol. 84, pp. 95-101.

Rubenstein, E.A., and G.V. Coelho, "Mental Health and Be-
  1970   havioral Sciences: One Federal Agency's Role in
            the Behavioral Sciences," <u>American Psycholo-</u>
            <u>gist</u>, vol. 25, pp. 517-523.

Sawyer, J., and M.F. Friedell, "The Interaction Screen:
  1965   An Operational Model for Experimentation on Inter-
            personal Behavior," <u>Behavioral Science</u>, vol. 10,
            pp. 446-459.

Scheflen, A.E., "Human Communication: Behavioral Programs
  1968   and Their Integration in Interaction," <u>Behavioral</u>
            <u>Science</u>, vol. 13, pp. 44-53.

Schein, E.H., and G.L. Lippitt, "Supervisory Attitudes To-
  1966   ward the Legitamacy of Influencing Subordinates,"
            <u>Journal of Applied Behavioral Science</u>, vol. 2,
            pp. 199-209.

Shepard, H.A., "Personal Growth Laboratories: Toward An
  1970   Alternative Culture," <u>Journal of Applied Behav-</u>
            <u>ioral Science</u>, vol. 6, pp. 259-266.

Shuman, L., et al., <u>A Model for Estimating Hospital Costs</u>,
  1971   Research Series No. 8, Blue Cross of Western
            Pennsylvania, June.

Tannenbaum, A.S., "An Event Structure Approach to Power and
  1962   to the Problem of Power Compatibility," <u>Behav-</u>
            <u>ioral Science</u>, vol. 7, pp. 315-331.

Ulrich, R.E., <u>Control of Human Behavior</u>, Glenview, Ill.:
  1966   Scott, Foresman & Co.

Winn, A., "Social Change in Industry: From Insight to
  1966   Implementation," <u>Journal of Applied Behavioral</u>
            <u>Science</u>, vol. 2, pp. 170-183.

Part 11.

MANAGEMENT: HISTORICAL BACKGROUND

Ackoff, R.L. (ed.), Progress in Operations Research, Vol.
1961   1, N.Y.: John Wiley & Sons.

Ackoff, R.L., and M. Sasieni, Fundamentals of Operations
1968   Research, N.Y.: John Wiley & Sons.

Andrews, K.R., "Toward Professionalism in Business Manage-
1969   ment," Harvard Business Review, vol. 47,
            March-April, pp. 50-51.

Ansoff, H.I., "The Firm of the Future," Harvard Business
1965   Review, September-October, pp. 162ff.

Applewhite, P.B., Organizational Behavior, Englewood
1965   Cliffs, N.J.: Prentice-Hall.

Argyris, C., Integrating the Individual and the Organiza-
1964   tion, N.Y.: John Wiley & Sons.

Aronofsky, J.S., Progress in Operations Research, Vol. III,
1969   N.Y.: John Wiley & Sons.

Beckett, J.A., Management Dynamics: The New Synthesis,
1971   N.Y.: McGraw-Hill.

Beer, S., Cybernetics and Management, N.Y.: John Wiley
1959   & Sons.

Beer, S., Management Science: The Business Use of Opera-
1967   tions Research, Garden City, N.Y.: Doubleday.

Bennett, J.B., and R.L. Weiher, "The Well-Read Manager,"
1972   Harvard Business Review, vol. 50, July-August,
            pp. 134-146.

Bennion, E.G., "Econometrics for Management," Harvard
1961   Business Review, March-April, pp. 100-112.

Bennis, W.G., Changing Organizations, N.Y.: McGraw-Hill.
1966

Bennis, W.G., K.D. Benne, and R. Chin, <u>The Planning of</u>
1969   <u>Change</u>, N.Y.: Holt, Rinehart & Winston.

Bennis, W.G., "Chairman Mac in Perspective," <u>Harvard</u>
1972   <u>Business Review</u>, vol. 50, September-October,
            pp. 140-149.

Berelson, B. (ed.), <u>The Behavioral Sciences Today</u>, N.Y.:
1963   Basic Books.

Blake, R.R., and J.S. Mouton, <u>Group Dynamics: Key to</u>
1961   <u>Decision Making</u>, Houston: Gulf Publishing.

Boulding, K.E., "General System Theory--The Skeleton of a
1956   Science," <u>Management Science</u>, April, pp.
            202-205.

Broehl, W.G., Jr., "Insights into Business & Society,"
1966   <u>Harvard Business Review</u>, May-June.

Burnham, J., <u>The Managerial Revolution</u>, N.Y.: The John
1941   Day Company.

Carzo, R., Jr., and J.N. Yanouzas, <u>Formal Organization: A</u>
1967   <u>Systems Approach</u>, Homewood, Ill.: Richard D.
            Irwin.

Churchman, C.W., "Managerial Acceptance of Scientific Re-
1964   commendations," <u>California Management Review</u>,
            Fall, pp. 31-38.

Churchman, C.W., and A.H. Schainblatt, "The Research and
1965   the Manager: A Dialectic of Implementation,"
            <u>Management Science</u>, vol. 11, February, pp.
            B69-B87.

Curcuru, E.H., and J.H. Healey, "The Multiple Roles of the
1972   Manager," <u>Business Horizons</u>, August, vol. 15,
            pp. 15-24.

Cyert, R.M., and J.G. March, <u>A Behavioral Theory of the</u>
1963   <u>Firm</u>, Englewood Cliffs, N.J.: Prentice-Hall.

Dale, E., The Great Organizers, N.Y.: McGraw-Hill.
    1960

Dale, E., Readings in Management, N.Y.: McGraw-Hill.
    1965

Dale, E., Organization,N.Y.: American Management Associa-
    1967   tion Press.

Dale, W., "Some Foundations of Organization Theory," Cali-
    1959   fornia Management Review, Fall, pp. 71-77.

Dantzig, G.B., "Management Science in the World of Today
    1967   and Tomorrow," Management Science, vol. 13,
                February, pp. C107-111.

Davis, K., "Evolving Models of Organizational Behavior,"
    1968   Academy of Management Journal, March.

Dearden, J.,and J. Lastavica, "New Directions in Operations
    1970   Research," Financial Executive, October,
                pp. 24-33.

Donnelly, J.H., Jr., J.L. Gibson, and J.M. Ivancevich,
    1971   Fundamentals of Management, Functions,
                Behavior, Models, Austin, Texas: Business
                Publications.

Drucker, P.F., "Long Range Planning: Challenge to Manage-
    1959   ment Science," Management Science, April,
                pp. 238-249.

Drucker, P.F., The Age of Discontinuity, N.Y.: Harper &
    1968   Row.

Drucker, P.F., "Management's New Role," Harvard Business
    1969   Review, November-December.

Dutton, J.M., and R.E. Walton, "Operational Research and
    1964   the Behavioral Sciences'," Operational Research
                Quarterly, vol. 15, pp. 207-217.

Eddy, W.B., W.W. Burke, V.A. Dupre, and O. South, Behavioral
    1969   Science and the Manager's Role, Los Angeles:
                NTL Learning Resources Corp.

Etzioni, A., A Comparative Analysis of Complex Organiza-
1961   tions, N.Y.: Free Press.

Ewing, D.W., "The Knowledge of an Executive," Harvard Busi-
1964   ness Review, March-April, pp. 91-100.

Fayol, H., General and Industrial Administration, London:
1949   Sir Isaac Pitman & Sons.

Feeney, G.J., "Time Sharing, Management, and Management
1967   Science," Management Science, vol. 13, Feb-
           ruary.

Feigenbaum, E., and J. Feldman (eds.), Computers and Thought,
1963   N.Y.: McGraw-Hill.

Ferber, R.C., and G. Fisk, "The Role of the Subconscious in
1967   Executive Decision-Making," Management Science,
           vol. 13, April.

Ferguson, L.L., "How Social Science Research Can Help
1966   Management," California Management Review,
           Summer, pp. 3-10.

Filippo, E.B., "Integrative Schemes in Management Theory,"
1968   Journal of the Academy of Management, vol. 11,
           March, pp. 91-98.

Filley, A.C., and R.J. House, Managerial Process and Organi-
1969   zational Behavior, Glenview, Ill.: Scott,
           Foresman and Co.

Frey, M.W. (ed), New Developments in Management and Organi-
1971   zation Theory, Amherst, Mass.: Eastern Aca-
           demy of Management, University of Massachu-
           setts.

Friedmann, J., "A Conceptual Model for Analysis of Planning
1967   Behavior," Administrative Science Quarterly,
           vol. 12, September, pp. 225-252.

Frederick, W.C., "The Next Development in Management: A
1963   General Theory," Journal of the Academy of
           Management, September.

Fulmer, R.M., "Profiles of the Future: The Management of
1972   Tomorrow," Business Horizons, vol. 15,
            August, pp. 5-13.

Galbraith, J.K., The New Industrial State, Boston:
1967   Houghton Mifflin.

George, C.S., Jr., The History of Management Thought,
1968   Englewood Cliffs, N.J.: Prentice-Hall.

Giffin, W.C., Introduction to Operations Engineering,
1971   Homewood, Ill.: Richard D. Irwin.

Good, I.J., "How Rational Should a Manager Be?" Management
1962   Science, vol. 88, July, pp. 383-393.

Gordon, P.J., "Transcend the Current Debate on Administra-
1965   tive Theory," in Management in Perspective,
            edited by W.E. Schlender, W.G. Scott, and A.C.
            Filley, Boston: Houghton Mifflin, pp. 5-18.

Graves, R.L., and P. Wolfe, Recent Advances in Mathematical
1963   Programming, N.Y.: McGraw-Hill.

Greenwood, W.T., Management and Organizational Behavior
1965   Theories, Cincinnati: South-Western Publish-
            ing.

Greenwood, W.T., Business Policy: A Management Audit
1967   Approach, N.Y.: Macmillan.

Greiner, L.E., "Evolution and Revolution as Organizations
1972   Grow," Harvard Business Review, vol. 50,
            July-August, pp. 37-47.

Groff, G.K., and J.F. Muth, Operations Management: Selected
1969   Readings, Homewood, Ill.: Richard D. Irwin.

Gruber, W.H., and J.S. Niles, "Put Innovation in the Organi-
1972   zation Structure," California Management
            Review, vol. 14, Summer, pp. 29-36.

Haimann, T., W.G. Scott, Management in the Modern Organi-
1970   zation, Boston: Houghton Mifflin Company

Haire, M. (ed.), <u>Organization Theory in Industrial Practice</u>,
1962   N.Y.:   John Wiley & Sons.

Haire, M., "The Social Sciences and Management Practices,"
1964   <u>California Management Review</u>, Summer, pp. 3-10.

Heany, D.F., "Is TIMS Talking to Itself?" <u>Management</u>
1965   <u>Science</u>, December, pp. B146-B155.

Helmstadter, G.C., <u>Research Concepts in Human Behavior</u>,
1970   N.Y.:   Appleton-Century-Crofts.

Herrmann, C.C., and J.F. Magee, "'Operations Research' for
1953   Management," <u>Harvard Business Review</u>, vol.
            31, July-August.

Hertz, D.B., "Mobilizing Management Science Resources,"
1965   <u>Management Science</u>, vol. 11, January, pp. 361-
            368.

Hicks, H.G., <u>The Management of Organizations: A Systems</u>
1972   <u>and Human Resources Approach</u>, 2nd edition,
            N.Y.:   McGraw-Hill.

Hillier, F.S., and G. J. Lieberman, <u>Introduction to Opera-</u>
1967   <u>tions Research</u>, San Francisco: Holden-Day.

Hollomon, J.H., "Technology in the United States: Issues
1972   and Options for the 1970's," <u>Technology Re-</u>
            <u>view</u>, vol. 74, June, pp. 10-22.

Hollomon, J.H., "Technology in the United States: The
1972   Options Before Us," Part II, <u>Technology Review</u>,
            vol. 74, July-August, pp. 32-42.

Keller, S., <u>Beyond the Ruling Class</u>, N.Y.:   Random House.
1963

Kolasa, B.J., <u>Introduction to Behavioral Science for Business</u>,
1969   N.Y.:   John Wiley & Sons.

Koontz, H., "The Management Theory Jungle," <u>Journal of the</u>
1961   <u>Academy of Management</u>, December.

Koontz, H. (ed.), Toward a Unified Theory of Management,
1964   N.Y.: McGraw-Hill.

Koontz, H., and C. O'Donnell, Principles of Management, 4th
1968   ed., N.Y.: McGraw-Hill.

Kuhn, T.S., The Structure of Scientific Revolutions, Chicago:
1962   The University of Chicago Press.

Larson, R.L., "How to Define Administrative Problems," Har-
1962   vard Business Review, vol. 40, January-February,
            pp. 68-80.

Leavitt, H.J., and T.L. Whisler, "Management in the 1980's,"
1958   Harvard Business Review, vol. 36, pp. 41-48.

Likert, R., New Patterns of Management, N.Y.: McGraw-Hill.
1961

Litterer, J.A., Organizations: Structure & Behavior, N.Y.:
1963   John Wiley & Sons.

Litterer, J.A., The Analysis of Organizations, N.Y.: John
1965   Wiley & Sons.

Luthans, F., Contemporary Readings in Organizational Be-
1972   havior, N.Y.: McGraw-Hill.

Machlup, F., "Theories of the Firm: Marginalist, Behavioral,
1967   Managerial," The American Economic Review,
            vol. 57, March, pp. 1-33.

March, J.G., and H.A. Simon, Organizations, N.Y.: John
1958   Wiley & Sons.

McFarland, D.E., Management, Principles and Practices,
1970   London: Collier-Macmillan.

McGregor, D., The Professional Manager, N.Y.: McGraw-Hill.
1967

McGregor, D., "An Uneasy Look at Performance Appraisal,"
1972   Harvard Business Review, vol. 50, September-
            October, pp. 133-139. (Originally printed in
            Harvard Business Review in 1957.)

Mee, J.F., *Management Thought in a Dynamic Economy*, N.Y.:
1963   New York University Press.

Merrill, H.F. (ed.), *Classics in Management*, N.Y.:   American
1960   Management Association Press.

Mills, C.W., *The Power Elite*, N.Y.:   Oxford University
1956   Press.

Moore, F.G. (ed.), *A Management Sourcebook*, N.Y.:   Harper
1964   & Row.

Morris, W.T., *The Analysis of Management Decisions*, Home-
1964   wood, Ill.:   Richard D. Irwin.

Morris, W.T., "Intuition and Relevance," *Management*
1967   *Science*, vol. 14, December, pp. B157-B165.

Morris, W.T., *Management Science*, Englewood Cliffs, N.J.:
1968   Prentice-Hall.

Newman, W.H., C.E. Summer, and E. K. Warren, *The Process*
1967   *of Management*, Englewood Cliffs, N.J.:
              Prentice-Hall.

Plane, D.R., and G.A. Kochenberger, *Operations Research for*
1972   *Managerial Decisions*, Homewood, Ill.:   Richard
              D. Irwin.

Raia, A.P., "Organizational Development--Some Issues and
1972   Challenges," *California Management Review*,
              Vol. 14, Summer, pp. 13-20.

Roberts, E.B., "Industrial Dynamics and the Design of
1963   Management Control Systems," *Management Tech-*
              nology, vol. 3, December, pp. 100-118.

Rosenzweig, J.E., "Managers and Management Scientists (Two
1967   Cultures)," *Business Horizons*, vol. 10,
              Vall, pp. 79-86.

Sayles, L., *Managerial Behavior*, N.Y.:   McGraw-Hill.
1964

Sayles, L., "Whatever Happened to Management?" <u>Business</u>
    1970   <u>Horizons</u>, April.

Schellenberger, R.E., <u>Managerial Analysis</u>, Homewood, Ill.:
    1969   Richard D. Irwin.

Scott, W.G., "Organization Theory: An Overview and an
    1961   Appraisal," <u>Journal of the Academy of Manage-</u>
                <u>ment</u>, April.

Scott, W.G., <u>Organization Theory</u>, Homewood, Ill.:   Richard
    1967   D. Irwin.

Scott, W.G., and T.R. Mitchell, <u>Organization Theory: A</u>
    1972   <u>Structural and Behavioral Analysis</u>, Homewood,
                Ill.: Richard D. Irwin.

Seen, P., "What is Behavioral Science--Notes Toward a
    1966   History," <u>Journal of the History of the Be-</u>
                <u>havioral Sciences</u>, vol. 2, pp. 107-122.

Simon, H.A., <u>Administrative Behavior</u>, N.Y.: Macmillan.
    1958

Simon, H.A., and A. Newell, "Heuristic Problem Solving,"
    1958   <u>Operations Research</u>, vol. 6, January, pp.
                1-10.

Sonthoff, H., "What is the Manager?" <u>Harvard Business Re-</u>
    1964   <u>view</u>, November-December, pp. 24-36, 188ff.

Starr, M.K. (ed.), <u>Executive Readings in Management Science</u>,
    1965   N.Y.: Macmillan.

Starr, M.K., "Planning Models," <u>Management Science</u>, vol.
    1966   13, December, pp. B115-B142.

Starr,M.K., <u>Management: A Modern Approach</u>, N.Y.: Harcourt
    1971   Brace Jovanovich.

Suojanen, W.W., "Management Theory: Functional and Evolu-
    1963   tionary," <u>Academy of Management Journal</u>,
                March, pp. 7-17.

Taylor, F.W., The Principles of Scientific Management,
1911   N.Y.: Harper & Brothers.

Teichroew, D., An Introduction to Management Science:
1964   Deterministic Models, N.Y.: John Wiley & Sons.

Tilles, S., "How to Evaluate Corporate Strategy," Harvard
1963   Business Review, vol. 41, July-August.

Tilles, S., "The Manager's Job--A Systems Approach," Har-
1963   vard Business Review, vol. 41, January-
            February, pp. 78-81.

Tomb, J.W., "A New Way to Manage--Integrated Planning and
1962   Control," California Management Review, vol.
            4, pp. 57-62.

Torgersen, P.E., and I.T. Weinstock, Management: An
1972   Integrated Approach, Englewood Cliffs, N.J.:
            Prentice-Hall.

Tracy, L., "Postscript to the Peter Principle," Harvard
1972   Business Review, vol. 50, July-August, pp.
            65-71.

Veinott, A.F., Jr. (ed.), Mathematical Studies in Manage-
1965   ment Science, N.Y.: Macmillan.

Wadia, M.S., The Nature and Scope of Management, Atlanta,
1966   Ga.: Scott, Foresmen & Co.

Wagner, H.M., "Practical Slants on Operations Research,"
1963   Harvard Business Review, May-June, pp. 61-71.

Wagner, H.M., Principles of Operations Research: With
1969   Applications to Managerial Decisions, Englewood
            Cliffs, N.J.: Prentice-Hall.

Wagner, H.M., Principles of Management Science: With Appli-
1970   cations to Executive Decisions, Englewood
            Cliffs, N.J.: Prentice-Hall.

Ways, M., "Tomorrow's Management: A More Adventurous Life
1966   in a Free-Form Corporation," Fortune, July 1.

Part 12.

ANALYTICAL MODELS

Acheson, E.D., and M.S. Feldstein, "Duration of Stay in Hos-
1964   pital for Normal Maternity Care," British Medi-
        cal Journal, vol. 2, no. 5401, pp. 95-99.

Aoki, M., Optimization of Stochastic Systems, N.Y.:
1967   Academic Press.

Bainbridge, L., et al., "Study of Real-Time Human Decision
1968   Making Using a Plant Simulator," Operational
        Research Quarterly, vol. 19, April, pp. 91-106.

Balintfy, J.L., "A Stochastic Model for the Analysis and
1960   Prediction of Admissions and Discharges in
        Hospitals," in Management Sciences: Models and
        Techniques, vol. 2, New York: Pergamon Press,
        pp. 288-299.

Balintfy, J.L., Outline of a Census Predictor Model for
1965   General Hospitals, Research Paper No. 16, New
        Orleans,La.: Computer Systems Research, Tulane
        University.

Balintfy, J.L., and A. Prekopa, "Nature of Random Variation
1966   in the Nutrient Composition of Means," Health
        Services Research, vol. 1, Fall, pp. 148-169.

Bartholomew, D.T., Stochastic Models for Social Processes,
1967   N.Y.: John Wiley & Sons.

Bartlett, M.S., An Introduction to Stochastic Processes,
1966   Cambridge, Mass.: Cambridge University Press.

Bashshur, R., et al., "The Application of Three-Dimensional
1970   Analogue Models to the Distribution of Medical
        Care Facilities," Medical Care, vol. 8, Septemb-
        er-October, pp. 395-407.

Beenhakker, H.L., "Multiple Correlation--A Technique for
1963   Prediction of Hospital Bed Needs," Operations
        Research, vol. 11, pp. 824-839.

Bithell, J.F., "A Class of Discrete-Time Models for the
1969   Study of Hospital Admission Systems," Operations
        Research, vol. 17, January-February, pp. 48-69.

Blumberg, M., "DPF Concept Helps Predict Bed Needs," The
1961   Modern Hospital, vol. 97, no. 6, pp. 75-81.

Boulden, J.B., and E.S. Buffa, "Corporate Models: On
1970   Line, Real Time Systems," Harvard Business Review,
        vol. 48, July-August, pp. 65-83.

Buff, J.H., et al., "Application of New Decision Analysis
1968   Techniques to Investment Research," Financial
        Analysts Journal, vol. 24, November, pp. 123-128.

Bursk, E.C., New Decision Making Tools for Managers,
1963   Cambridge, Mass.: Harvard University Press.

Catassi, C.A., and E.L. Peterson, "The Blood Inventory Con-
1967   trol System--Helping Blood Bank Management Through
        Computerized Inventory Control," Transfusion,
        vol. 7, February, pp. 60-69.

Chiang, C.L., "An Index of Health Statistics, Mathematical
1965   Models," Vital and Health Statistics, United
        States Department of Health, Education and Wel-
        fare, Series 2, No. 5, May.

Crowston, W., and G.L. Thompson, "Decision CPM: A Method
1967   of Simultaneous Planning, Scheduling and Control
        of Projects," Operations Research, vol. 15,
        May, pp. 407-426.

Cushing, B.E., "Application Potential of Integer Program-
1970   ming," Journal of Business of the University of
        Chicago, vol. 43, October, pp. 457-467.

Das, R.S., "Service Gate Information and Prediction of De-
1964   mand for Hospital Services," Opsearch (India),
        vol. 1, no. 3, pp. 141-150.

Davies, R.L., "Facilities and Equipment for Health Ser-
1966   vices," Milbank Memorial Fund Quarterly, vol. 49,
        July, pp. 249-269.

Denardo, E.V., "Separable Markovian Decision Problems,"
    1968   Management Science, vol. 14, March, pp. 451-462.

Derman, C., "On Sequential Decision and Markov Chains,"
    1962   Management Science, vol. 9, no. 1, pp. 16-24.

Devos, H., and R.A. Farmer and Associates, Inc., Practical
    1968   Techniques and Policies for Inventory Control,
            N.Y.: American Institute of Certified Public
            Accountants.

Elston, R.C., and J.C. Pickrel, "A Statistical Approach to
    1963   Ordering and Usage Policies for a Hospital Blood
            Bank," Transfusion, vol. 3, p. 1126.

Elston, R.C., and J.C. Pickrel, "Guides to Inventory Levels
    1965   for a Hospital Blood Bank Determined by Elec-
            tronic Computer Simulation," Transfusion, vol. 5,
            September, pp. 465-470.

Enrick, N.L., Inventory Management: Installation, Operation,
    1968   and Control, San Francisco, Calif.: Chandler
            Publishing Co.

Fahs, I.J., et al., "Indicators of Need for Health Care Per-
    1971   sonnel: The Concept of Need, Alternative Meas-
            ures Employed to Determine Need, and a Suggested
            Model," Medical Care, vol. 9, March-April, pp.
            144-151.

Feldstein, M., "Improving the Use of Hospital Maternity
    1965   Beds," Operational Research Quarterly, vol. 16,
            no. 1, pp. 65-76.

Feldstein, P.J., and J.J. German, "Predicting Hospital
    1965   Utilization: An Evaluation of Three Approaches,"
            Inquiry, vol. 2, no. 1, pp. 13-36.

Flagle, C.D., "Operations Research in a Hospital," Opera-
    1960   tions Research and Systems Engineering, Balti-
            more, Md.: The Johns Hopkins Press, pp. 763-785.

Flagle, C.D., "Operations Research in the Health Services,"
    1962   Operations Research, vol. 10, no. 5, pp. 591-
            603.

Flagle, C.D., W.H. Huggins, and R.H. Ray, <u>Operations Re-</u>
1960   <u>search and Systems Engineering</u>, Baltimore, Md.:
       The Johns Hopkins Press.

Flagle, C.D., and J.P. Young, "Applications of Operations
1966   Research and I.E. to Problems of Health Service
       Hospitals and Public Health," <u>Journal of Indus-</u>
       <u>trial Engineering</u>, vol. 17, no. 11, pp. 609-613.

Foster, F.G., "Batched Queuing Processes," <u>Operations Re-</u>
1964   <u>search</u>, vol. 12, May-June, pp. 441-449.

Fulkerson, D.R., "Expected Critical Path Lengths in PERT
1962   Networks," <u>Operations Research</u>, vol. 10, Novem-
       ber-December, pp. 808-817.

Glover, F., "Management Decision and Integer Programming,"
1969   <u>Accounting Review</u>, vol. 44, April, pp. 300-303.

Gorry, G.A., and G.O. Barnett, "Experience with Model of
1968   Sequential Diagnosis," <u>Computer and Biomedical</u>
       <u>Research</u>, vol. 1, May, pp. 490-507.

Grubbs, F.E., "Attempts to Validate Certain PERT Statis-
1962   tics or 'Picking on PERT'," <u>Operations Research,</u>
       vol. 10, November-December, pp. 912-915.

Gue, R.L., and M.E. Thomas, <u>Mathematical Methods in Opera-</u>
1968   <u>tions Research</u>, N.Y.: Macmillan.

Gustafson, G.H., "Length of Stay: Prediction and Explana-
1968   tion," <u>Health Services Research</u>, vol. 3, Spring,
       pp. 12-34.

Hess, I., and K.S. Srikantan, "Some Aspects of the Pro-
1966   bability Sampling Technique of Controlled
       Selection," <u>Health Services Research</u>, vol. 1,
       no. 1, pp. 8-52.

Horvath, W.J., "The Systems Approach to the National
1966   Health Problem," <u>Management Science</u>, vol. 12,
       June, pp. B 391-B 396.

Hsieh, R.K.C., "Evaluation of Formal Communications Systems
1966   in a Hospital," Health Services Research, vol. 1,
        Winter, pp. 222-234.

Hurlbert, E.L., and A.R. Jones, "Blood Bank Inventory Con-
1964   trol," Transfusion, vol. 4, no. 2, pp. 126-133.

Jackson, R.R.P., et al., "Appointments Systems in Hospitals
1964   and General Practice," Operational Research
        Quarterly, vol. 15, no. 3, pp. 219-237.

Jansson, B., "Choosing a Good Appointment System--A Study
1966   of Queues of the Type D/M/I," Operations Research,
        vol. 14, March-April, pp. 292-312.

Jelinek, R.C., "A Structural Model for the Patient Care
1967   Operation," Health Services Research, vol. 2,
        Fall-Winter, pp. 226-242.

Jennings, J.B., "Hospital Blood Bank Whole Blood Inventory
1967   Control," Technical Report No. 27, Cambridge,
        Mass.: M.I.T. Press, December.

Jensen, R.E., "Sensitivity Analysis and Integer Linear
1968   Programming," Accounting Review, vol. 43, July,
        pp. 425-446.

Johnson, W.D., and G.G. Koch, "Analysis of Qualitative
1970   Data: Linear Functions," Health Services
        Research, vol. 5, Winter, pp. 358-369.

Ledley, R.S., "Computer Aids to Clinical Treatment Evalua-
1967   tion," Operations Research, vol. 15, July-
        August, pp. 591-778.

Lincoln, T.L., and R.D. Parker, "Medical Diagnosis Using
1967   Bayes Theorem," Health Services Research, vol.
        2, Spring, pp. 34-45.

Lincoln, T.L., and G.H. Weiss, "A Statistical Evaluation of
1964   Recurrent Medical Examinations," Operations Re-
        search, vol. 12, March-April, pp. 187-205.

Management Operating System--Inventory Management and Mater-
    ials Planning-Detail, I.B.M., No. E20-0050.

Management Operating System--Forecasting Materials, Planning
    and Inventory Management--General, I.B.M.,
    No. E20-0031.

Miller, R.W., "How to Plan and Control with PERT," Harvard
    1962   Business Review, vol. 40, no. 2, pp. 93-104.

Moon, J.E., "Computerized Pharmacy Systems Solves Hospital
    1969   Drug Inventory Problems," Modern Hospital, vol.
    113, November, p. 118+.

Navarro, V., et al., "A Stochastic and Deterministic Model
    1970   of Medical Care Utilization," Health Services
    Research, vol. 5, Winter, pp. 342-357.

Newell, D.J., "Problems in Estimating the Demand for Hos-
    1964   pital Beds," Journal of Chronic Disease, vol.
    17, August, pp. 749-760.

Odoni, A.R., "Finding the Maximal Gain for Markov Decision
    1969   Processes," Operations Research, vol. 17, Sep-
    tember, pp. 857-860.

Ortiz, J., and J. Parker, "Birth-Life-Death Model for Plan-
    1971   ning and Evaluation of Health Services Programs,"
    Health Services Research, vol. 6, Summer, pp.
    120-143.

Pett, L.B., "Operational Research and Health Services,"
    1965   Canadian Journal of Public Health, vol. 56,
    November, pp. 457-461.

Pike, M.C., et al., "Analysis of Admissions to a Casualty
    1963   Ward," British Journal of Preventive Social
    Medicine, vol. 17, October, pp. 172-176.

Pocock, J.W., "PERT As An Analytical Aid for Program Plan-
    1962   ning--Its Payoff and Problems," Operations
    Research, vol. 10, December, pp. 893-903.

Resh, M., <u>Mathematical Programming of Admissions Scheduling</u>
  1967 <u>in Hospitals</u>, Doctoral Dissertation, Johns Hopkins
      University (Dept. of O.R. and I.E.).

Robinson, G.H., "Hospital Admission Scheduling Control,"
  1965 <u>Report No. HFT-65-4, Human Factors in Technology</u>
      <u>Research Group</u>, Berkley, Calif.: University of
      California, Department of Industrial Engineering.

Robinson, G.H., et al., "Prediction of Hospital Length of
  1966 Stay," <u>Health Services Research</u>, vol. 1, Winter,
      pp. 287-300.

Robinson, G.H., et al., "The Physician as an Estimator of
  1966 Hospital Stay," <u>Human Factors</u>, vol. 8, pp.201+.

Rockwell, T.H., et al., "Inventory Analysis as Applied to
  1962 Hospital Whole Blood Supply and Demand," <u>Journal</u>
      <u>of Industrial Engineering</u>, vol. 13, no. 2, pp.
      109-114.

Roman, D.D., "The PERT System: An Appraisal of Program
  1962 Evaluation Review Technique," <u>Academy of Manage-</u>
      <u>ment Journal</u>, vol. 5, April, pp. 57-65.

Rustagi, J.S., "Dynamic Programming Model of Patient Care,"
  1968 <u>Mathematical Bioscience</u>, vol. 3, August, pp.
      141-149.

Singer, S., <u>A Stochastic Model of Variation of Categories</u>
  1961 <u>of Patients Within a Hospital</u>, Doctoral Disser-
      tation, Johns Hopkins University, I.E. Dept.

Smalley, H.E., et al., "Hospital Bed Study," <u>Hospital</u>
  1963 <u>Management Systems Society Research</u>, <u>Pub. No. 1</u>,
      <u>HMSS</u>, Birmingham, Al.: University of Alabama
      Press.

Soriano, A., "Comparison of Two Scheduling Systems," <u>Oper-</u>
  1966 <u>ations Research</u>, vol. 14, May-June, pp. 388-397.

Stallings, R.A., "Hospital Adaptations to Disaster: Flow
  1970 Models of Intensive Technologies," <u>Human Organi-</u>
      <u>zation</u>, vol. 29, Winter, pp. 294-302.

Sullivan, D.F., "Conceptual Problems in Developing an Index
1966   of Health," Vital and Health Statistics, Nat-
        ional Center for Health Statistics, Public Health
        Service Publication No. 1000, Series 2, No. 17,
        Washington, D.C.: Government Printing Office,
        May.

Thierauf, R.J., Decision Making Through Operations Research,
1970   N.Y.: John Wiley & Sons.

Thompson, J., et al., "Predicting Requirements for Mater-
1963   nity Facilities," Hospitals, February.

Vandell, R.F., "Management Evolution in the Quantitative
1970   World," Harvard Business Review, vol. 43,
        pp. 83-92.

Warner, H.R., et al., "Mathematical Approach to Medical
1961   Diagnosis: Application to Congenital Heart
        Disease," Journal of the American Medical Associ-
        ation, vol. 117, July 22, pp. 177-183.

Weckwerth, V.E., "Determining Bed Needs from Occupancy and
1966   Census Figures," Hospitals, vol. 40, January 1,
        pp. 52-54.

White, L.S., "Bayes Markovian Decision Models for Multi-
1967   period Reject Allowance Problem," Operations
        Research, vol. 15, September, pp. 857-865.

Wolfe, H., A Multiple Assignment Model for Staffing Nursing
1964   Units, Doctoral Dissertation, Johns Hopkins
        University, Department of O.R. and I.E.

Woolf, C.R., et al., "The Use of Program Evaluation and
1968   Review Technique (PERT) in the Decision and Con-
        trol of a Medical Research Project," Computers
        and Biomedical Research, vol. 2, October, pp.
        176-186.

Young, J.P., "Administrative Control of Multiple Channel
1966   Queuing Systems with Parallel Input Streams,"
        Operations Research, vol. 14, January-February,
        pp. 145-156.

Part 13.

SIMULATION MODELS

Adlinger, G.R., "Business Games--Play One!" Harvard Busi-
1958   ness Review, vol. 36, March, pp. 115-125.

Alutto, J.A., and J.A. Belasco, "A Typology for the Parti-
1972   cipation in Organizational Decision Making,"
        Administrative Science Quarterly, vol. 17,
        March, pp. 117-125.

Au, T., et al., Hospital System Design Simulation, Hospital
1970   System Design Group, Pittsburgh, Pa.,: Carnegie-
        Mellon University Press, August.

Babb, E.M., and L.M. Eisgraber, Management Games for Teach-
1966   ing and Research, Chicago: Educational Methods.

Babb, E.M., et al., "The Potential of Gaming Methods in
1966   Research," The Journal of Business, vol. 49,
        p. 456.

Baisuck, A., and W. A. Wallace, "Computer Simulation Ap-
1970   proach to Enrollment Projection in Higher Edu-
        cation," Socio-Economic Planning Sciences,
        vol. 4, September, pp. 365-381.

Banks, M.H., "Gaming and Simulation in International Re-
1968   lations," Political Studies, vol. 16, February,
        pp. 1-17.

Barish, N.N., and F. H. Siff, "Operational Gaming with Ap-
1969   plication to a Stock Market," Management
        Science, vol. 15, June, pp. 530-541.

Basil, D.C., et al., Executive Decision Making Through
1965   Simulation, London: Prentice-Hall International,
        pp. 213, 405.

Bass, B.M., Business Gaming for Organizational Research,"
1964   Management Science, vol. 10, April, pp. 545-556.

Bass, B.M., and J.A. Vaughan, Training in Industry: The
  1966   Management of Learning, Belmont, Calif.:
            Wadsworth Publishing Co.

Bauer, R.A., and R.D. Buzzell, "Mating Behavioral Science
  1964   and Simulation," Harvard Business Review, vol.
            42, September-October, pp. 116-124.

Beaver, M.W., "Maternity Unit Admissions Policy and the
  1970   Use of Simulations," British Journal of Pre-
            ventive and Social Medicine, vol. 24, August,
            pp. 169-176.

Berman, R.R., "Simulation as a Problem Solving Technique,"
  1967   American Society Civil Engineers Proc., vol. 93,
            March, pp. 21-45.

Bohn, G., and C.G. Richie, "Learning by Simulation: The
  1970   Validation of Disaster Simulation," Journal
            of the Kansas Medical Society, vol. 71, Novem-
            ber, pp. 418-425.

Boocock, S.S., "Simulation Games Today," Educational
  1968   Technology, vol. 8, pp. 7-10.

Bradley, M.N., "Using GPSS Simulation in Operations Re-
  1969   search," Journal of Systems Management, vol.
            20, January, pp. 18-21.

Brenner, M.E., "Relation Between Decision Making Penalty
  1965   and Simulation Sample Size for Inventory Sys-
            tems," Operations Research, vol. 13, May, pp.
            433-443.

Broad, E., Jr., "Planning a Multilevel Car Park," Indus-
  1969   trial Engineering, September, pp. 17-23.

Brundage, M., and J.L. Livingstone, "Simulation on a Time-
  1969   Sharing Computer Utility System," Accounting
            Review, vol. 44, July, pp. 539-545.

Burch, J., "Business Games and Simulation Techniques,"
  1969   National Association of Accountants Journal,
            vol. 51, December, pp. 49-55.

Burling, J.M., "Discrete Simulation: New Tool for Control
  1970   and System Design," Control Engineering, vol.
            17, May, pp. 77-85.

Chorafas, D.N., Systems and Simulation, New York: Academic
  1965   Press.

Cohen, K., and E. Rhenman, "The Role of Management Games
  1961   in Education and Research," Management Science,
            vol. 7, January, pp. 131-166.

Conway, R.W., "Some Tactical Problems in Digital Simula-
  1963   tion," Management Science, vol. 10, October,
            pp. 47-61.

Crecine, J.P., "Computer Simulation Model of Municipal
  1967   Budgeting," Management Science, vol. 13, July,
            pp. 786-815.

Cremens, J.E., "Trends in Simulation," Computer and Auto-
  1968   mation, vol. 17, January, pp. 44-48.

Crowston, W., and G.L. Thompson, "Decision CPM: A Method
  1967   of Simultaneous Planning, Scheduling and
            Control of Projects," Operations Research, vol.
            15, May, pp. 407-427.

Cushing, B.E., "Application Potential of Integer Program-
  1970   ming," Journal of Business of the University
            of Chicago, vol. 43, October, pp. 457-465.

Dale, A.G., and C.K. Klasson, Business Gaming: A Survey of
  1964   American Collegiate Schools of Business, Austin,
            Texas: The University of Texas, Bureau of
            Business Research.

Danziger, E.N., et al., "The Administrator's Role and Res-
  1967   ponsibilities in Computer Mechanization,"
            Hospital Administration, vol. 12, Spring, pp.
            24-33.

Demski, J., "Second Conference on Applications of Simula-
  1969   tion," Datamation, vol. 15, February, pp. 85+.

Dill, W.R., and N. Doppelt, "The Acquisition of Experience
1963   in a Complex Management Game," Management
         Science, vol. 10, October.

Duke, R.D., and R.L. Meier, "Gaming Simulation for Urban
1966   Planning," American Institute of Planners
         Journal, vol. 32, January, pp. 3-17.

Dunn, L.R., "Application of Simulation Rationale for Evalu-
1969   ation," Naval Engineering Journal, vol. 81,
         February, pp. 79-87.

Durham, R.C., and R. Buchan, "Using Computer Simulation
1970   Modeling to Reduce Hospital Waiting Lines,"
         Hospital Topics, vol. 48, April, pp. 47-52.

Easton, A., "Simulation Model of Pricing Decisions," Jour-
1969   nal of Systems Management, vol. 20, May, pp.
         14-21.

Ebner, D., "Technique of Simulation," Journal of Systems
1970   Management, vol. 21, February, pp. 19-23.

Eitzen, D.S., and N.R. Yetman, "Managerial Change, Longe-
1972   vity, and Organizational Effectiveness," Ad-
         ministrative Science Quarterly, vol. 17, March,
         pp. 110-116.

Elincki, R., "R.O.I. Simulations for Investment Decisions,"
1970   National Association of Accountants Journal,
         vol. 15, February, pp. 37-41.

Elveback, L., et al., "Simulation of Mathematical Models
1965   for Public Health Problems," Public Health
         Reports, vol. 80, December, pp. 1067-1076.

Emshoff, J., and R. Sisson, Design and Use of Computer
1970   Simulation Models, N.Y.: Macmillan.

Enrick, N.L., "Management Simulation of Inventory Systems,"
1965   Indiana Conference Board, vol. 66, May, pp.
         26.32.

Feldstein, M.S., "Improving the Use of Hospital Maternity
1965   Beds," Operational Research Quarterly, vol.
          16, March, pp. 65-76.

Fetter, R.B., and J.D. Thompson, "The Simulation of Hospital
1965   Systems," Operations Research, vol. 13, Septem-
          ber-October, pp. 689-711.

Fine, G., and P.F.McIsaac, "Simulation of a Time-Sharing
1966   System," Management Science, vol. 12, February,
          pp. 180-194.

Fishman, G.S., "Allocation of Computer Time in Comparing
1968   Simulation Experiments," Operations Research,
          vol. 16, March, pp. 280-295.

Flagle, C.D., "Role of Simulation in Health Services,"
1970   American Journal of Public Health, vol. 60,
          December, pp. 2386-2394.

Forrester, J.W., "A Deeper Knowledge of Social Systems,"
1969   Technology Review, vol. 71, April, pp. 21-31.

Forrester, J.W., Urban Dynamics, Cambridge, Mass.: The
1969   M.I.T. Press.

Gearon, J.D., "Labor vs. Management: A Simulation Game,"
1966   Social Education, October, pp. 421-22.

Geisler, M.A., and W.A. Steger, "The Combination of Alter-
1963   native Research Techniques in Logistics Systems
          Analysis," Management Technology, vol. 3,
          May, pp. 68-76.

Giffin, S.F., The Crisis Game: Simulating International
1965   Conflict, Garden City, N.Y.: Doubleday.

Glatt, M.A., "The Design of an Engineering Management
1966   Game," Operations Research, B19A.

Goetz, B.E., "Synthesis of Several Simulation Techniques,"
1969   Management Science, vol. 15, June, pp. 506-511.

Gordon, G., and K. Zelin, "A Simulation Study of Emergency
1968   Ambulance Service in New York City," Technical
            Report No. 320-2935, I.B.M. Corp., March.

Goslin, L.N., "Decisions for Growth: Analysis by Simula-
1969   tion," Operational Research Quarterly, vol.
            20, June, pp. 187-197.

Graham, R.G., and C. F. Gray, Business Games Handbook, N.Y.:
1969   American Management Association Press.

Gray, C., "P.E.R.T. Simulation: A Dynamic Approach to the
1969   PERT Technique," Journal of Systems Management,
            vol. 20, March, pp. 18-25.

Gross, D., and A. Soriano, "Effect of Reducing Leadtime in
1969   Inventory Levels--Simulation Analysis," Manage-
            ment Science, vol. 16, October, pp. 61-76.

Handyside, A.J., and D. Morris, "Simulation of Emergency
1967   Bed Occupancy," Health Services Research, vol.
            2, Fall-Winter, pp. 287-297.

Haussman, R.K.D., "Waiting Time as an Index of Quality of
1970   Nursing Care," Health Services Research, vol.
            5, Summer, pp. 92-105.

Hearn, C.R., and J.M. Bishop, "Computer Model Simulating
1970   Medical Care in Hospital," British Medical'
            Journal, vol. 3, August 15, pp. 396-399.

Hertz, D.B., "Risk Analysis in Capital Investment,"
1964   Harvard Business Review, vol. 42, January-
            February, pp. 95-106.

Hespos, R.F., "Simulation as an Aid to Staffing a Customer
1968   Service Function," Management Technology, vol.
            3, December, pp. 160-166.

Hickok, W.H., A Bibliography of Research Studies on Games
1967   and Simulations, Portland, Ore.: Northwest
            Regional Education Laboratory.

Hoggatt, A.C., "Measuring the Cooperativeness of Behavior in
   1967   Quantity Variation Duopoly Games," Behavioral
            Science, vol. 12, pp. 109-121.

Holland, E.P., "Principles of Simulation," American Behav-
   1965   ioral Scientist, vol. 9, September, pp. 6-10.

Howland, D., "A Hospital System Model," Nursing Research,
   1963   vol. 12, Fall, pp. 232-236.

Hunter, J., "Experimental Designs for Computer Simulation
   1970   Experiments," Management Science, vol. 16,
            March, pp. 422-434.

Hunter, R.F., and J.E. Schnee, "Long Range Planning in
   1966   Mental Health," Management Science, vol. 12,
            August, pp. B519-B524.
Hutte, H., "Decision-Making in a Management Game," Human
   1965   Relations, vol. 18, no. 1, pp. 5-20.

Jackson, R.R.P., et al., "Appointments Systems in Hospitals
   1964   and General Practice," Operational Research
            Quarterly, vol. 15, September, pp. 219-237.

Kaufman, G.M., and R. Penchansky, "Simulation Study of Union
   1968   Health and Welfare Funds," Industrial Manage-
            ment Review, vol. 10, Fall, pp. 41-60.

Kenney, J.L., "Clinical Study of the Use of Simulation
   1967   Model," Journal of Industrial Engineering,
            vol. 18, January, pp. 30-35.

Kesling, G., "Project Analysis by Computer Simulation,"
   1970   Journal of Systems Management, vol. 21, March,
            pp. 14-21.

Khemakhem, A., "A Simulation of Management-Decision Behav-
   1968   ior," The Accounting Review, vol. 18, July,
            pp. 522-534.

Kibbee, J.M., et al., Management Games, N.Y.: Reinhold
   1961   Publishing Co.

Kidera, E.H., and J.M. Hoff, "Simulation: Management Tool
1968   in Decision Making," Automation, vol. 15,
          February, pp. 83-88.

Klasson, C.R., "Business Gaming: A Progress Report,"
1964   Academy of Management Journal, vol. 8, Septem-
          ber, pp. 175-188.

Kleijnen, J., et al., "The Use of Multiple Ranking Proce-
1972   dures to Analyze Simulations of Management
          Systems: A Tutorial," Management Science,
          vol. 18, February, pp. B245-B257.

Krasnow, H.S., and R. Merikallio, "The Past, Present and
1964   Future of General Simulation Languages," Manage-
          ment Science, vol. 11, November.

Lahdenmaki, T., and L. Sulonen, "Simulation Techniques in
1970   Hospital Planning," World Hospitals, vol. 6,
          October, pp. 193-196.

LeGrande, E., "The Development of a Factory Simulation
1963   System Using Actual Operating Data," Manage-
          ment Technology, vol. 3, May, pp. 1-18.

Lerner, E., "Simulating a Cash Budget," California Manage-
1968   ment Review, vol. 11, Winter, pp. 79-86.

Lewin, A.Y., and W.L. Weber, "Management Game Teams in Edu-
1969   cation and Organization Research: An Experi-
          ment in Risk Taking," Journal of the Academy
          of Management, vol. 12, March, pp. 49-58.

Ludwig, R.H., "Simulation with Decision Tables," Journal
1968   of Data Management, vol. 6, January, pp. 20-24.

McKenney, J.L., Simulation Gaming for Management Develop-
1967   ment, Boston, Mass.: Graduate School of Busi-
          ness Administration, Harvard University.

McMillan, C., and R.F. Gonzalez, Systems Analysis: A Com-
1965   puter Approach to Decision Models, Homewood,
          Ill.: Richard D. Irwin.

Meir, R.C., et al., Simulation in Business and Economics,
    1969   Englewood Cliffs, N.J.: Prentice-Hall.

Naylor, T.H., "Bibliography on Simulation and Gaming,"
    1969   Computing Reviews, January.

Naylor, T.H., and J.M. Finger, "Verification of Computer
    1967   Simulation Models," Management Science, vol.
                14, October, pp. 92-106.

Packer, A.H., "Simulation and Adaptive Forecasting as Ap-
    1967   plied to Inventory Control," Operations Re-
                search, vol. 15, July, pp. 660-679.

Perna, G., "Inventory Systems Simulation--A Case Study,"
    1968   National Association of Accountants Journal,
                vol. 49, July, pp. 50-54.

Philippakis, A., "Mathematical Analysis U.S. Simulation
    1969   Methods," Journal of Systems Management, vol.
                20, May, pp. 28-31.

Porter, J.C., et al., "The Use of Simulation as a Pedago-
                gical Device," Technical Paper No. 091465,
                Management Science Center, Wharton School of
                Finance and Commerce, University of Pennsyl-
                vania.

Proceedings and Report of Conference on a Health Manpower
    1970   Simulation Model, vol. 1 and 11, U.S. Depart-
                ment of Health, Education and Welfare, Public
                Health Service, National Institute of Health,
                Washington, D.C.: Government Printing Office.

Rath, G.J., et al., "Simulation of a Hematology Department,"
    1970   Health Services Research, vol. 5, Spring, pp.
                25-35.

Ricciardi, F.M., et al., Top Management Decision Simulation,
    1967   the AMA Approach, N.Y.: American Management
                Association Press.

Robinson, G.H., "Computer Simulation of Hospital Patient
    1968   Scheduling System," Health Services Research,
                vol. 3, Summer, pp. 130-141.

Robinson, G.H., et al., "A Simulation Model for the Evalua-
    1964   tion of Scheduling Decision Rules for Hospital
              Elective Admissions," Research Report HFT-64-
              5T, The Human Factors in Technology Research
              Group, Berkley,Calif.: University of California
              Press.

Sagar, R.G., and L.K. Dick, "Computer Simulation of Ambul-
    1971   ance Services: A Decision-Making Aid for the
              Administrator, Canadian Hospital, vol. 48, May,
              pp. 23+.

Salazar, R.C., and S.K. Sen, "Simulation Model of Capital
    1968   Budgeting Under Uncertainty," Management Sci-
              ence, vol. 15, December, pp. B 161-B 179.

Savas, E., "Simulation and Cost-Effectiveness Analysis of
    1969   New York's Emergency Ambulance Service," Man-
              agement Science, vol. 15, August, pp. B 608-
              B 627.

Schmidt, J.W., and R.E. Taylor, Simulation and Analysis of
    1970   Industrial Systems, Homewood, Ill.:   Richard
              D. Irwin.

Schwartz, H., "Wise up! That Computer is Just a Giant
    1972   Moron," The New York Times, Sunday, March 19.

Shao, D.M., A Stochastic Model for the Study of the Waiting
    1970   Time of Non-Emergency Patients in a Hospital
              Admission System, Buffalo, N.Y.: State Univer-
              sity of New York at Buffalo.

Shonick, W., "A Stochastic Model for Occupancy-Related Ran-
    1970   dom Variables in General-Acute Hospitals,"
              Journal of American Statistical Association,
              vol. 65, December, pp. 1474-1500.

Shubik, M., "Gaming: Costs and Facilities," Management
    1968   Science, vol. 14, July, pp. B629-B 660.

Sihler, W.W., "Toward Better Management Control Systems,"
    1971   California Management Review, vol. 14, Winter,
              pp. 33-49.

Smith, R.D., and P.S. Greenlaw, "Simulation of a Psycholo-
1967   gical Decision Process in Personnel Selection,"
        Management Review, vol. 56, April, pp. 409-419.

Smith, V.L., "Effect of Market Organization on Competitive
1964   Equilibrium," Quarterly Journal of Economics,
        vol. 78, May, pp. 181-202.

Starr, M.K., Management: A Modern Approach, N.Y.: Harcourt
1971   Brace Jovanovich.

Symonds, G.H., "A Study of Management Behavior by Use of
1964   Competitive Business Games," Management Science,
        vol. 11, September, pp. B 135-B 153.

Thies, J.B., "Computer Modeling and Simulation: A Manage-
1970   ment Tool for Systems Definition and Analysis,"
        Financial Executive, vol. 38, September, pp.
        20-27.

Thompson, J.D., and R.B. Fetter, "Use of Computer Simula-
1963   tion Techniques in Predicting Requirements for
        Maternity Facilities," Hospitals, vol. 37,
        February 16, pp. 45-49, 132.

Thorelli, H.B., "Integrated Use of Simulations in Management
1964   Education," Personnel Journal, vol. 40, no. 2,
        pp. 67-71.

Torgerson, P.E., "Introducing Queuing Concepts: A Simula-
1967   tion Approach," Journal of Industrial Engineer-
        ing, vol. 18, May, pp. 328-333.

Vance, G.R., "Inventory Simulation: Concepts, Implementa-
1968   tion and Benefits," Management Accounting,
        vol. 49, July, pp. 50-54.

Vance, S., Management Decision Simulation, N.Y.: McGraw-
1961   Hill.

Vance, S.C., and C.F. Gray, "Use of a Performance Evaluation
1967   Model for Research in Business Gaming," Journal
        of the Academy of Management, vol. 10, March,
        pp. 27-37.

Williams, W.J., et al., "Simulation Modeling of a Teaching
    1967   Hospital Outpatient Clinic," <u>Hospitals</u>, vol.
             41, November 1, pp. 71-75.

Wing, P., "Automated System for Scheduling Admissions,"
    1967   <u>Hospital Management</u>, vol. 104, October, p.53.

Wing, P., and G.H. Robinson, "Computer Programs for Simula-
    1966   ting Hospital Scheduling System," <u>Report No.
             HFT-66-1, Human Factors in Technology Research
             Group</u>, Berkley, Calif.: University of Califor-
             nia.

Zoll, A.A., III, <u>Dynamic Management Education</u>, Reading,
    1969   Mass.: Addison-Wesley, pp. 368-500.

Part 14.

TOWARD A PERSPECTIVE

Andersen, R., and O.W. Anderson, A Decade of Health Ser-
1967   vices: Social Survey Trends in Use and Ex-
            penditure, Chicago, Ill.: University of
            Chicago Press.

Badgley, R.F., and S. Wolfe, Doctors' Strike, Medical Care
1967   and Conflict in Saskatchewan, N.Y.: Atherton.

Barnett, G.O., "Can Computers Reduce Manpower Needs?"
1971   Hospitals, vol. 45, August 16, pp. 55-57.

Barzun, J., The House of Intellect, N.Y.: Harper & Row.
1959

Barzun, J., Science: The Glorious Entertainment, N.Y.:
1964   Harper & Row.

Battistella, R.M., and T.P. Weil, Health Care Organization:
1971   Bibliography and Guidebook, Washington, D.C.:
            Association of University Programs in Hospital
            Administration, April.

Bauer, R.A. (ed.), Social Indicators, Cambridge, Mass.:
1966   M.I.T. Press.

Bell, D., and I. Kristol (eds.), Capitalism Today, N.Y.:
1971   Basic Books.

Bennis, W.G., and P.E. Slater, The Temporary Society, N.Y.:
1968   Harper & Row.

Boguslaw, R., The New Utopians - A Study of System Design
1965   and Social Change, Englewood Cliffs, N.J.:
            Prentice-Hall.

Boulding, K.E., The Meaning of the 20th Century: The Great
1964   Transition, N.Y.: Harper & Row.

Bronowski, J., Science and Human Values, N.Y.: Julian
1956   Messner.

Bruner, J.S., <u>On Knowing</u>, Cambridge, Mass.: Harvard Univer-
1962   sity Press.

Bryant, J., <u>Health and the Developing World</u>, Ithaca, N.Y.:
1969   Cornell University Press.

Buckley, W. (ed.), <u>Modern Systems Research for the Behav-</u>
1968   <u>ioral Scientist</u>, Chicago, Ill.: Aldine.

Clark, K.B., <u>Dark Ghetto</u>, N.Y.: Harper & Row.
1965

Cloward, R.A., and F.F. Piven, "A Strategy to End Poverty,"
1966   <u>Nation</u>, vol. 202, May 2, pp. 510-517.

Coe, R.M. (ed.), <u>Planned Change in the Hospital: Case</u>
1970   <u>Studies of Organizational Behavior</u>, N.Y.:
            Praeger.

Cohen, W.J., "Social Indicators, Statistics for Public
1968   Policy," <u>American Statistician</u>, vol. 22,
            October, pp. 14-16.

Crichton, M., <u>Five Patients</u>, N.Y.: Alfred A. Knopf.
1970

Cumming, Elaine, <u>Systems of Social Regulation</u>, N.Y.:
1968 Atherton.

Dahl, R.A., and C.E. Lindblom, <u>Politics, Economics, and</u>
1953   <u>Welfare</u>, N.Y.: Harper & Row.

Davis, F., "Uncertainty in Medical Prognosis, Clinical and
1960   Functional," <u>American Journal of Sociology</u>,
            vol. 66, pp. 41-47.

de Beauvoir, S., <u>The Coming of Age</u>, N.Y.: G.P. Putnam's
1972   Sons.

deHartog. J., <u>The Hospital</u>, N.Y.: Atheneum.
1964

Donabedian, A., "Social Responsibility for Personal Health
1971   Services: An Examination of Basic Values,"
            Inquiry, vol. 8, June, pp. 3-19.

Drucker, P.F., "Management's New Role," Harvard Business
1969   Review, vol. 47, November-December, pp. 49-54.

Drucker, P.F., Technology, Management and Society, N.Y.:
1970   Harper & Row.

Dubos, R., Man, Medicine, and Environment, N.Y.: Praeger.
1968

Duff, R.S., and A.B. Hollingshead, Sickness and Society,
1968   N.Y.: Harper & Row.

Ehrenreich, B., and J. Ehrenreich, The American Health
1970   Empire, N.Y.: Random House.

Eller, J.C., "The Denominational Hospital: Past, Present
1969   and Future," Hospital Progress, vol. 50,
            September, pp. 79-81.

Ellul, J., The Technological Society, N.Y.: Alfred A.
1964   Knopf.

Etzioni, A., and E. Etzioni, Social Change, N.Y.: Basic
1964   Books.

Fairweather, G.W., Methods for Experimental Social Innova-
1968   tion, N.Y.: John Wiley & Sons.

Fein, R., The Doctor Shortage: An Economic Diagnosis,
1967   Washington, D.C.: The Brookings Institution.

Fein, R., "Medical Care Needs in the Coming Decade,"
1969   Bulletin of the New York Academy of Medicine,
            vol. 45, March, pp. 255-270.

Feldstein, M.S., The Rising Cost of Hospital Care,
1971   Washington, D.C.: Information Resources Press.

Forrester, J.W., Principles of Systems, Cambridge, Mass.:
1967   M.I.T. Press.

Forrester, J.W., Urban Dynamics, Cambridge, Mass.: M.I.T.
1969   Press.

Forsyth, G.C., and D.G. Thomas, "Models for Financially
1971   Healthy Hospitals," Harvard Business Review,
              vol. 49, August, pp. 106-117.

Fraser, R.D., "Health and General Systems of Financing
1972   Health Care," Medical Care, vol. 10, July-
              August, pp. 345-356.

Freidson, E., Professional Dominance: The Social Structure
1970   of Medical Care, N.Y.: Atherton Press.

Fuchs, V.R., "Health Care and the United States Economic
1972   System," The Milbank Memorial Fund Quarterly,
              vol. 2, April, Part I, pp. 211-237.

Fuchs, V.R., The Service Economy, N.Y.: National Bureau of
1968   Economic Research.

Gardner, J.W., Excellence, N.Y.: Harper & Row.
1961

Gardner, J.W., Self-Renewal, N.Y.: Harper & Row.
1963

Georgopolous, B.S., and F.C. Mann, The Community General
1962   Hospital, N.Y.: Macmillan.

Georgopoulos, B.S. (ed.), Organization Research on Health
1972   Institutions, Ann Arbor, Mich.: Institute for
              Social Research, University of Michigan.

Geyman, J.P., The Modern Family Doctor and Changing Medical
1971   Practice, N.Y.: Appleton-Century-Crofts.

Ginzberg, E., Urban Health Services: The Case of New York,
1971   N.Y.: Columbia University Press.

Ginzberg, E., D.L. Hiestand, and B.G. Reubens, The Plural-
1965   istic Economy, N.Y.: McGraw-Hill.

Glaser, W.A., <u>Paying the Doctor: Systems of Remuneration</u>
1970   <u>and Their Effects</u>, Baltimore: The Johns Hop-
            kins Press.

Glazer, B.G., and A. Strauss, <u>Awareness of Dying</u>, Chicago:
1965   Aldine.

Glazer, N., and D.P. Moynihan, <u>Beyond the Melting Pot</u>,
1963   Cambridge, Mass.: M.I.T. Press.

Goodrich, C.E., M. Olendzki, and G. Reader, <u>Welfare Medical</u>
1970   <u>Care: An Experiment</u>, Cambridge, Mass.:
            Harvard University Press.

Goodrich, C., M. Olendzki, and A.F. Crocetti, "Hospital-
1972   based Comprehensive Care: Is it a Failure?"
            <u>Medical Care</u>, vol. 10, July-August, pp.
            363-368.

"Graduate Education for Hospital Administration," <u>Hospital</u>
1967   <u>Administration</u>, vol. 12, Fall.

Grube, E.F., "Hospital Mergers," <u>Hospitals</u>, vol. 45, May,
1971   pp. 45-48.

Gruen, V., <u>The Heart of Our Cities: The Urban Crisis:</u>
1964   <u>Diagnosis and Cure</u>, N.Y.: Simon & Schuster.

<u>Guidelines for Health Services R & D: Hospital Mergers</u>,
1972   National Center for Health Services Research
            and Development, Department of Health, Educa-
            tion, and Welfare, February.

<u>Guidelines for Health Services R & D: Shared Services</u>,
1972   National Center for Health Services Research
            and Development, Department of Health, Educa-
            tion, and Welfare, February.

Haar, C.M., and P.A. Lewis, "Where Shall the Money Come
1970   From?" <u>The Public Interest</u>, vol. 18, Winter,
            pp. 101-112.

Hamilt, M.W., "Problems and Trends to be Faced as Allied
1971   Health Professions Evolve," <u>Hospital Manage-</u>
            <u>ment</u>, vol. 112, August, p. 20.

Harrington, M., The Other America, N.Y.: Macmillan.
  1962

Harrington, M., The Accidental Century, Baltimore, Md.:
  1965   Penguin Books.

Heilbroner, R.L., The Limits of American Capitalism, N.Y.:
  1966   Harper & Row.

Heilbroner, R.L., et al., In the Name of Profit, Garden
  1972   City, N.Y.: Doubleday.

Hershey, N., "New Directions in Licensure of Health
  1971   Personnel," Economic and Business Bulletin,
              vol. 24, pp. 22-35.

Hofstadter, R., Social Darwinism in American Thought,
  1955   Boston, Mass.: Beacon Press.

Hofstadter, R., Anti-Intellectualism in American Life,
  1963   N.Y.: Alfred A. Knopf.

Hook, S. (ed.), Human Values and Economic Policy, N.Y.:
  1967   New York University Press.

Horty, J.F., "Michigan Statute Tightens Trustee Control of
  1969   Care," Modern Hospital, vol. 112, January,
              pp. 48-50.

Horty, J.F., "Changing Practices Pose Legal Problems for
  1969   Hospitals," Modern Hospital, vol. 112, March,
              pp. 62-64.

Horvath, W., "Need for Estimating the Influence of Techno-
  1968   logical and Social Changes on Future Health
              Facility Requirements," Health Services Re-
              search, vol. 3, Spring, pp. 3-9.

Hughes, E., Men and Their Work, Glencoe, Ill.: Free Press.
  1958

Jacobs, J., The Death and Life of Great American Cities,
  1961   N.Y.: Modern Library.

Jaeger, B.J., "Government and Hospitals: A Perspective on
1972   Health Politics," Hospital Administration,
          vol. 17, Winter, pp. 39-50.

Jencks, C., and D. Riesman, The Academic Revolution, N.Y.:
1968   Doubleday.

Kahn, A.J., Theory and Practice of Social Planning, N.Y.:
1969   Russell Sage Foundation.

Kahn, H., and A.J. Wiener, The Year 2000, N.Y.: Macmillan.
1967

Kaluzny, A.D., J.E. Veney, J.T. Gentry, and J.B. Sprague,
1971   "Scalability of Health Services: An Empirical
          Test," Health Services Research, Fall, pp.
          214-223.

Keniston, K., The Uncommitted: Alienated Youth in American
1965   Society, N.Y.: Harcourt Brace.

Kerr, C., The Uses of the University, Cambridge, Mass.:
1963   Harvard University Press.

Knowles, J.H. (ed.), Hospitals, Doctors, and the Public
1965   Interest, Cambridge, Mass.: Harvard University
          Press.
Knowles, J.H. (ed.), The Teaching Hospital, Cambridge, Mass.:
1966   Harvard University Press.

Knowles, J.H. (ed.) Views of Medical Education and Medical
1968   Care, Cambridge, Mass.: Harvard University
          Press.

Krech, D., "Controlling the Mind Controllers," Think, vol.
1966   32, July-August, pp. 3-7.

Kuhn, T., The Structure of Scientific Revolutions, Chicago,
1962   Ill.: University of Chicago Press.

Lee, P.R., "Role of the Federal Government in Health and
1968   Medical Affairs," New England Journal of
          Medicine, vol. 279, November 21, pp. 1139-1147.

Lindblom, C.E., "Economics and the Administration of Na-
1964   tional Planning," Public Administration Re-
             view, vol. 25, December, pp. 274-283.

Lubove, R., The Professional Altruist, Cambridge, Mass.:
1965   Harvard University Press.

Lynd, R.S., Knowledge For What? Princeton, N.J.: Prince-
1967   ton University Press.

Magraw, R.M., Ferment in Medicine, Philadelphia, Pa.:
1966   Saunders and Company.

McKeown, T., Medicine in Modern Society, N.Y.: Hafner
1966   Publishing.

Mead, M., "Neighborhoods and Human Needs," EKISTICS,
1966   vol. 21, February.

Mechanic, D., Mental Health and Social Policy, Englewood
1969   Cliffs, N.J.: Prentice-Hall.

Mechanic, D., "Problems in the Future Organization of Medi-
1970   cal Practice," Law and Contemporary Problems,
             vol. 35, pp. 233-251.

Mendelsohn, E.I., J.P. Swazey, and I. Taviss (eds.), Human
1971   Aspects of Biomedical Innovation, Cambridge,
             Mass.: Harvard University Press.

Mesthene, E.G. (ed.), Technology and Social Change,
1967   Indianapolis, Indiana: Bobbs-Merrill.

Mesthene, E.G., Technological Change: Its Impact on Man
1970   and Society, Cambridge, Mass.: Harvard Univer-
             sity Press.

Milio, N., "Health Care Organizations and Innovation,"
1971   Journal of Health and Social Behavior, vol.
             12, June, pp. 163-173.

Millis, J.S., A Rational Public Policy for Medical Education
1971   and its Financing, N.Y.: The National Fund
             for Medical Education.

Moss, A.R., et al., <u>Hospital Policy Decisions: Process and</u>
1966   <u>Action</u>, N.Y.:   J.P. Putnam's Sons.

Moynihan, D.P., <u>Maximum Feasible Misunderstanding: Commu-</u>
1969   <u>nity Action in the War on Poverty</u>, N.Y.:   The
            Free Press.

Muller, H.J., <u>Freedom in the Modern World</u>, N.Y.:   Harper
1966   & Row.

Muller, H.J., <u>The Children of Frankenstein</u>, Bloomington,
1970   Ind.:   Indiana University Press.

Mumford, E., <u>Interns: From Students to Physicians</u>,
1970   Cambridge, Mass.:   Harvard University Press.

Mumford, L., <u>The Myth of the Machine: Technics and Human</u>
1967   <u>Development</u>, N.Y.:   Harcourt, Brace and World.

"The Nation's Health: Some Issues", <u>The Annals of the</u>
1972   <u>American Academy of Political and Social</u>
            <u>Science</u>, vol. 399, January.

Perloff, H.S., and L. Wingo, Jr. (eds.), <u>Issues in Urban</u>
1968   <u>Economics</u>, Baltimore, Maryland: Johns Hopkins
            Press.

Pomrinse, S.D., "To What Degree are Hospitals Publicly
1969   Accountable?" <u>Hospitals</u>, vol. 43, pp. 41-44.

Popper, H. (ed.), <u>Trends in New Medical Schools</u>, N.Y.:
1967   Grune and Stratton.

Proshansky, H. (ed.), <u>Environmental Psychology-Man and His</u>
1970   <u>Physical Setting</u>, N.Y.:   Holt, Rinehart and
            Winston.

Rafkind, F.B., <u>Health Maintenance Organizations: Some</u>
1972   <u>Perspectives</u>, Chicago, Ill.:   Blue Cross
            Association, May.

Rayack, E., <u>Professional Power and American Medicine: The</u>
1967   <u>Economics of the American Medical Association</u>,
            Cleveland: World Publishing Company.

Remmling, G.W., <u>Road to Suspicion</u>, N.Y.: Appleton-Century-
1967   Crofts.

Richmond, J.B., <u>Currents in American Medicine</u>, Cambridge,
1969   Mass.: Harvard University Press.

Roemer, M.I., and D.M. DuBois, "Medical Costs in Relation
1969   to the Organization of Ambulatory Care,"
           <u>New England Journal of Medicine</u>, vol. 280,
           May 1, pp. 988-994.

Roemer, M.I., D.M. DuBois, and S.W. Rich, <u>Health Insurance</u>
1970   <u>Plans: Studies in Organizational Diversity</u>,
           Los Angeles: School of Public Health, U.C.L.A.

Roemer, M.I., and J.W. Friedman, <u>Doctors in Hospitals:</u>
1971   <u>Medical Staff Organization and Hospital Per-</u>
           <u>formance</u>, Baltimore, Md.: Johns Hopkins Press.

Rogers, E.M., <u>Diffusion of Innovations</u>, N.Y.: The Free
1962   Press.

Rosenbloom, R.S., and J.R. Russell, <u>New Tools for Urban</u>
1971   <u>Management</u>, Cambridge, Mass.: Graduate School
           of Business Administration, Harvard University.

Rusalem, H., <u>Coping with the Unseen Environment</u>, N.Y.:
1972   Columbia University Press.

Schottland, C.I., <u>The Social Security Program in the United</u>
1963   <u>States</u>, N.Y.: Appleton-Century-Crofts.

Selekman, B.M., <u>A Moral Philosophy for Management</u>, N.Y.:
1959   McGraw-Hill.

Simon, H.A., <u>Models of Man</u>, N.Y.: John Wiley & Sons.
1957

Snow, C.P., <u>The Two Cultures: A Second Look,</u> London:
1964   Cambridge University Press.

Somers, A.R., <u>Hospital Regulation: The Dilemma of Public</u>
1969   <u>Policy,</u> Princeton, N.J.: Industrial Relations
           Section, Princeton University.

Somers, A.R., "These are the Questions About Regulation.
1969   What King? How Much? By Whom? Why?" Modern
            Hospital, vol. 113, September, pp. 137-141.

Somers, A.R., "University Hospital: Future Role," Hospi-
1971   tals, vol. 45, November 16, pp. 41-53.

Somers, A.R., and H. Somers, Medicare and the Hospitals,
1967   Washington, D.C.: Brookings Institution.

Somers, H.M., and A.R. Somers, Doctors, Patients and Health
1961   Insurance, Washington, D.C.: Brookings
            Institution.

Sorokin, P.A., Social and Cultural Dynamics, N.Y.:
1962   Bedminster Press.

Starkweather, D.B., and S.J. Taylor, Health Facility Com-
1970   binations and Mergers: An Annotated Biblio-
            graphy, Chicago, Ill.: American College of
            Hospital Administrators

Stevens, R., American Medicine and the Public Interest,
1971   New Haven, Conn.: Yale University Press.

Taviss, I., "Futurology and the Problem of Values,"
1969   International Social Science Journal, vol. 21,
            pp. 574-584.

Taylor, G.R., The Biological Time Bomb, N.Y.: World
1968   Publishing.

Theobald, R., The Challenge of Abundance, N.Y.: C.N.
1961   Potter.

Theobald, R. (ed.), The Guaranteed Income: Next Step in
1966   Economic Evolution, N.Y.: Random House.

Titmuss, R.M., Essays on the Welfare State, New Haven:
1959   Yale University Press.

Todd, C.D., Jr., "Hospitals' Organizational Structure:
1971   Trend Toward the Corporate Form," Hospitals,
            vol. 45, September, pp. 55-59.

"Toward the Year 2000: Work in Progress," _Daedalus_,
1967   Summer.

Viguers, R.T., "Tomorrow's Voluntary Health Care System:
1969   The Challenge for the Hospital," _Hospital
           Progress_, vol. 50, June, pp. 68-71.

White, K.L., "Research in Medical Care and Health Service
1968   Systems," _Medical Care_, vol. 6, pp. 95-100.

Wildavsky, A., _The Politics of the Budgetary Process_,
1964   Boston: Little, Brown, and Co.

Wilensky, H.L., _Organizational Intelligence_, N.Y.:
1967   Basic Books.

Yablonski, L., _The Tunnel Back_, N.Y.: Macmillan.
1964

Young, M., _Rise of the Meritocracy, 1870-2033_, N.Y.:
1959   Random House.